PLANNING FOR THE NATION'S HEALTH

PLANNING FOR THE NATION'S HEALTH

A Study of Twentieth-Century Developments in the United States

GRACE BUDRYS

Contributions in Medical Studies, Number 19

GREENWOOD PRESS
New York • Westport, Connecticut • London

Library of Congress Cataloging-in Publication Data

Budrys, Grace, 1943–
  Planning for the nation's health.

  (Contributions in medical studies, ISSN 0886–8220 ;
no. 19)
  Bibliography: p.
  Includes index.
  1. Health planning—United States—History.
2. Medical policy—United States—History.   3. Social
medicine—United States—History.   I. Title.
II. Series.
  RA395.A3B83   1986   362.1'0973   86–12142

  ISBN 0–313–25348–X (lib. bdg. : alk. paper)

Library of Congress Catalog Card Number: 86–12142
ISBN: 0–313–25348–X
ISSN: 0886–8220

First published in 1986

Greenwood Press, Inc.
88 Post Road West, Westport, Connecticut 06881

Printed in the United States of America

The paper used in this book complies with the
Permanent Paper Standard issued by the National
Information Standards Organization (Z39.48–1984).

10 9 8 7 6 5 4 3 2 1

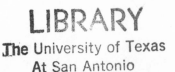

Contents

Tables

Preface

The research on which this volume is based began in response to an announcement in autumn 1981 by Department of Health and Human Services spokesmen that the health planning enterprise, particularly the funding supporting health systems agencies (HSAs), was to be phased out during the forthcoming year. Some HSAs have been phased out since then. However, the majority accommodated to the new social environment which decreed that health planning in its current form was an approach whose time had come and gone. Henceforth, planning was to be carried out according to the dictates of the marketplace.

As a sociologist interested in health care delivery arrangements, I wondered how the organizations involved would respond to such an overt threat to their existence. One of my primary concerns was finding out what would happen to the knowledge and experience accumulated by the health planning agencies, so I approached one such agency to discuss the possibility of my studying its day-to-day activities as a participant-observer.

The administration and governing board of the HSA, called the Urban HSA in the text, welcomed my interest in focusing on the knowledge and experience that had accrued. However, any references to my interest in the organization's response to the newly evolving hostile environment were regarded as morbid and totally unacceptable. Thus, we agreed that the question to be addressed would be: What have we learned from our experience with health planning? (For a description of the research site and an account of the course that the case study took throughout the period spent with the HSA, see the appendix.)

In attempting to answer this question, I quickly found that health planning had a far more complex history than I had realized. I also discovered that the steps leading to prevailing health planning arrangements were recorded in scattered bits and pieces. I began by reconstructing the origins of health planning for my own purposes (chapter 2). The effects of health planning efforts, both short term and long term, became the focus of chapter 3. The thinking that was responsible for the health planning proposals and programs that came into existence in the past is dealt with in chapter 4. Chapter 5 reviews the health planning literature of the past three decades, when health planning evaluation research evolved.

It is only after this background material is in place that I turn to the agency studied. While I employ a sociological perspective throughout, it is most explicit in the portion of the discussion devoted to the case study findings. However, since few sociologists have commented on health planning to date, I found no established sociological foundation upon which to build. Therefore, the discussion speaks to the ideas of political scientists and economists who have labored in this area. When I began this study, there also had been very little cross-disciplinary discussion on the topic of health planning between economists and political scientists. An interdisciplinary identification of "health services researcher," which emerged since that time, has already had integrating effects (via a journal, an association, annual meetings, and such). This development, however, has not caused many more sociologists to become interested in issues related to health planning. Accordingly, I hope, first, that this volume will stimulate the interest of a larger number of sociologists in the topic of health planning. Second, I hope that those health services researchers who are already familiar with much of this material will find that considering it from another, that is, sociological, perspective provokes fresh thought and reflection that will have a beneficial effect on the continuing effort to plan for the nation's health.

I wish to express my appreciation to the members of the HSA staff, who, unfortunately, must remain anonymous, for their generosity in welcoming me to participate in the work being done by the agency. I was permitted complete access to their files, went along on site visits, sat in on sessions in which staff reports were formulated, and so on. Both the consumer and provider representatives were also generous in finding the time to talk to me about their impressions of the HSA's performance. I am grateful to all of them.

Also, I wish to acknowledge the support of DePaul University in the form of research grants for 1983 and 1984. Finally, I am grateful to a number of friends and colleagues whose contribution goes well beyond their willingness to listen or to read material related to this particular research effort. This is especially true in the case of Dan Lortie, my husband, who has come to learn more about health planning than he ever intended.

PLANNING FOR THE NATION'S HEALTH

1

The Topic of Health Planning

A growing body of literature found under the rubric of health planning has come into existence since the late 1960s. While the concerns addressed by the health planning literature also fall under the topic headings of health policy and health care delivery, the latter headings are far broader in scope. Moreover, they typically discuss prevailing health care arrangements with the aim of analyzing the impact that such arrangements have on major health indicators, such as mortality and morbidity rates, utilization of health care services, or shifts in health behavior (for example, smoking or use of emergency rooms). In some instances, the effects that might be forthcoming from various alternative arrangements such as pre-paid care, increased co-payment, or reduction in certain basic resources (such as hospital beds or number of surgeons) are also considered. The health planning literature, by contrast, focuses primarily on proposals and programs aiming to alter the processes responsible for the design of the health care delivery system.

If an initial review of this literature does not result in the impression that it is a distinct topic, this may be because the health planning label has been superimposed on earlier works in order to place health planning in a larger historical context. Health planning emerged as an area of interest during the mid 1960s. Any earlier initiatives discussed under this rubric have been so designated retrospectively.

There have been no efforts to reach back to the nineteenth century, since the single most effective method of controlling disease prior to the twentieth century was recognized to be public sanitation. Successful planning efforts carried out by communities to address public sanitation problems are documented in the public health literature. Health care on the individual level prior to the twentieth century did not achieve nearly as much success. It was only toward the end of the nineteenth century that evidence began to accumulate indicating that "regular physicians'' were producing better results with their treatments than their many competitors who espoused a variety of explanations for illness and prescribed an equally diverse range of cures. It is not until the first decade of the twentieth century that success was achieved in more than 50 percent of the cases treated by regular physicians according to the oft-quoted statement by Lawrence Henderson:

I think it was about the year 1910 or 1912 when it became possible to say of the United States that a random patient with a random disease consulting a doctor chosen at random stood better than a fifty-fifty chance of benefiting from the encounter. (attributed by Gregg 1956, 13)

Thus, health planning can be distinguished from earlier concerns about health because it addresses problems associated with the delivery of health care to individuals for their distinctive health problems rather than for problems perceived to be common to all persons within the community. Once it became clear that the quality of health care could make a significant difference to the health of an individual, health care became a prized commodity. Initially, like many other scarce commodities, it was distributed according to the individual's ability to pay for it. However, as America became more prosperous and more workers had the wherewithal to purchase many kinds of commodities, health care began to be viewed as a right rather than a privilege. As a result, the government was drawn into the matter in order to facilitate a more equitable distribution of a valued commodity to which, it was decided, everyone was entitled.

The health planning body of literature has undergone a period of enormous expansion over the past few decades, which suggests that the topic has been increasing in salience, meaning there must be a high level of interest in altering the existing health care delivery system. "Otherwise why bother to plan?" (Feingold 1969; 807). There is no question that health care has emerged as an important social issue thought to deserve a great deal of public, professional, and legislative attention. Accordingly, massive amounts of time, effort, and money have been expended to address society's concerns about health care delivery in recent years. It is remarkable, therefore, that the sense of crisis about this topic does not abate (Wildavsky 1977). A majority of Americans (61%) currently consider the system to be in crisis (Andersen, Fleming, and Champney 1982). About three-quarters of the population thinks that major changes in the structure of the system are needed (Harris 1983; Iglehart 1984). According to the American Medical Association: "Public concern about health care costs has reached the highest level ever measured in an American Medical Association poll" ("Public Expresses Increased Concern . . . " 1984). How is it that the application of extensive effort and vast amounts of resources have seemingly been unable to produce a greater level of public satisfaction regarding the nation's health care system?

Since various steps have been taken in order to address public concerns, and few seem to have satisfied the public, the question that remains unanswered is: What changes would correct the flaws in the system that are responsible for the prevailing level of public dissatisfaction with current health care delivery arrangements? A wide range of opinion seems to exist regarding the likelihood that the kinds of alterations that would decrease public dissatisfaction can be effected. Some observers claim that significant change is unlikely no matter how much effort is expended on attempting to alter current health care delivery arrangements because the vested interests in the system are so entrenched (Alford 1975; Lipsky and Lounds 1976; West and Stevens 1976; Navarro 1976; Krause 1977; Vladek 1977; and Tannen 1980). Others believe that the problem is grounded in unrealistic expectations about medicine's abilities coupled with what seems to be an insatiable level of demand for health care (Wildavsky 1977). There are also those who believe that the expectations held by the American public are perfectly reasonable (Anderson 1985, 261). The few observers who believe that the organization of the health care delivery system can be improved seem to be fairly confident about it. This is the faction pointing out that the processes associated with earlier planning efforts were flawed, suggesting that if better processes could be developed, the problems associated with health care delivery could be greatly reduced if not totally resolved (Marmor and Morone 1980; Institute of Medicine 1981).

Moving along a dimension defined by expectations regarding the likelihood that the system can be altered, thereby resolving current problems, we find a number of observers occupying the middle ground. Immershein (1981) and Vladek (1977), for example, claim that the system lends itself to incrementalism and muddling through via minor modifications rather than revolutionary changes and that it will continue to perform accordingly. Feingold (1969) and Ginzberg (1969) argue that this is because the public is basically apathetic and has not demanded changes. Anderson (1968) predicted that changes would occur when society felt impelled to demand them. Under what circumstances changes will be demanded remains unclear. However, recent evidence from other sectors suggests that the public can be of two minds on a number of public issues—deeply dissatisfied about the state of social institutions in general but sufficiently satisfied personally—to allow the status quo to continue without demanding extensive change (Caplow 1982).

A possible explanation for the continuing level of public dissatisfaction with health care delivery arrangements is that earlier problems have been, to a large extent, satisfactorily resolved, but they have been replaced by newer, more complex problems. In fact, earlier solutions have contributed to creating new problems. Moreover, the larger context in which the system of health care delivery exists has not stood still. It has been changing at a pace that is more rapid than the health planning enterprise, as it was structured, could absorb. Another important contributing factor can be found in the rhetoric that frames discussion about health care delivery arrangements in the public media, which must rely on the scholarly press and government reports as their sources. One can find persons cited as experts arguing with unsettling frequency that the most recent attempts to address health sector problems, whatever they may be, are misguided and ineffective. Therefore, they argue, these efforts should be replaced with the particular mechanism (that is, incentive system, altered reimbursement schedule, and such) being promoted by that expert. It is no wonder that the public is convinced that the health sector is in a state of crisis. Added to the fact that the public is being confronted with conflicting assessments regarding the performance of the health care delivery system is the problem society is having absorbing and giving meaning to the technological advances being introduced in the sector. This is especially true of the awesome capability that medical technology has developed to sustain life, almost indefinitely, with all the ethical, financial, and social implications that have yet to be resolved (President's Commission for the Study of Ethical Problems . . . 1982). Lending greater credence to this point of view is the fact that closer examination of public opinion data reveals little public consensus about the nature of the crisis in health care. Perhaps there is no single factor and it is after all a crisis of confusion. Blendon and Altman (1984) call it a ''national schizophrenia.'' They also point out that while the public can readily identify a number of reasons for seeing a crisis in the health care sector, the public sees even more pressing problems in other sectors.

Why the public sense of crisis regarding health care arrangements does not abate, why there is so little agreement within the health care sector regarding a suitable approach for monitoring and controlling ongoing development, and why most observers of the system find so much to criticize can be better understood if one examines health planning in the broader framework provided by the passage of time. I will utilize a four-stage framework to organize the discussion to follow, the primary contribution of which is its focus on the changes that the definition of the problem regarding prevailing health care arrangements has undergone during the twentieth century. Health planning efforts were motivated by a different set of concerns during each of the four periods identified, all calling for a different set of solutions, which, in turn, have led to certain effects, initially considered desirable but which themselves proved to be problematic in later periods. The four stages are:

I. PRIVATE SECTOR HEALTH PLANNING

This phase begins at the turn of the century and ends in the late 1950s. The *quality* of health care was the dominant concern during this period.

II. THE INITIAL STAGE IN PUBLIC SECTOR HEALTH PLANNING

This is the period between the late 1950s and the early 1970s. It is during this time that *access to health care* emerged as the primary goal.

III.   THE ADVANCED STAGE IN PUBLIC SECTOR
HEALTH PLANNING

This period starts in the early 1970s and lasts to the end of the decade. During these years access to health care was edged out as the primary focus of concern by interest in *cost containment*.

IV.   RATIONALIZATION OF HEALTH PLANNING

This period begins around 1980 and is showing no signs of being supplanted by a new phase as yet. This is an era characterized by recognition of the fact that health care has become an industry and the hope that rationalization and centralization will result in greater *managerial efficiency*. If sufficient savings are not achieved, the specter of rationing looms in the shadows of current discussions. (Fuchs 1984; Aaron and Schwartz 1984)

This outline brings the focus to bear on one especially important fact: while each phase ushered in a new definition of the problem, the existing definition was not abandoned. Instead, the definitions have been cumulative. Currently, society is demanding that all of the earlier goals be met—the highest level of quality possible, equality of access, cost containment, and, finally, that this be accomplished efficiently (Luft and Frisvold 1979; Institute of Medicine 1980). Clearly, what has occurred is that with each successive phase, the goals have become more complicated and the means required to achieve them more difficult to specify. In fact, the latest definition of the problem sets forth an impossible task, that is, maximizing essentially contradictory aims with quality and access on one side and cost containment plus increased efficiency on the other. Adding to the complexity of this task is the fact that, to date, no one has been prepared to specify the extent of achievement that would constitute success with respect to each of these goals.

Before discussing the current situation further, I should point out that the most recent initiatives launched by the government have definitely not been identified as health planning programs. Indeed, the stated intent of government spokesmen is to dismantle the entire health planning enterprise. Nevertheless, for purposes of this discussion, I will treat these programs as health planning initiatives. Even though it is true that the steps taken by the government reduced the role played by those associated with health planning as it was conceived during the 1960s and 1970s, this is not because the need for planning is now thought to be unimportant. Rather, what has changed is the thinking regarding who is best suited to fulfill that responsibility. Thus, health planning is most assuredly taking place, albeit with an entirely new cast of participants who have brought with them a different set of goals, means, and planning methodologies.

In effect, the decisions being made at present regarding the operations of the health sector are not being identified as health planning by the authors of these plans; and it cannot be said that health planning, in the strictest sense, was taking place during the first half of the twentieth century. It is truly a product of the 1960s and 1970s in its conventional meaning. However, health planning is used here in the broadest sense possible in order to trace the thinking which led to each increment in the evolving design of the health care delivery system from the beginning of the century to the present.

There is another reason for including the most recent government initiatives in a review of health planning over the twentieth century. This decision lays the basis for considering the three main systems of social control society has at its disposal for overseeing the governance of major social institutions (Ellwood 1974; Mead 1977; Palmer 1979). These are professional, administrative, and market controls. To illustrate, the following shifts in social control have occurred within the health care sector during this century:

During phase I control over the health care system rested in the hands of the medical profession. This was the era of *professional control*.

Phase II was initiated on the assumption that physicians would be willing to share control on a voluntary basis with interested members of the public. Thus, we had a form of *administrative control grounded in voluntarism*.

In phase III administrative control was reinforced via stronger administrative planning guidelines, increased regulatory power invested in planning agencies, and a reduction in the role assigned to the "providers" of health care. In this form, we experienced *administrative control combined with regulation*.

Market control has been introduced during phase IV. Competition and consumer choice are central to this approach. (In actuality competition both for consumers' loyalty and dollars is constrained by reimbursement schedules administered by third party payers which, in turn, are heavily influenced by the reimbursement programs used by the federal government, especially the DRG Medicare reimbursement schedule. This will be discussed in greater detail later.)

In effect, a limited number of social control alternatives exists from which to choose. Clearly, over the past two or three decades, the representatives of society charged with the responsibility for making such choices have been casting about in an attempt to identify an acceptable approach which would satisfy the growing number of interested participants who have established a stake in the future development of the health care sector.

Focusing on the system of control that has existed at a particular time, the reasons explaining its emergence, and the circumstances under which shifts to an alternate system of control took place since the beginning of this century reveals the trends in thinking that are responsible for the pattern of evolution experienced by the health care sector (the subject of a substantial share of the discussion to follow). In fact, to some extent the perception of a crisis in the health care sector may be attributable to society's inability to find a combination of control mechanisms to produce a sense of confidence in this sector.

Accordingly, one of the major aims of this book is to focus on the structural shortcomings, as well as the benefits, of each form of social control over the health care sector that society has experienced to date. While I do not conclude by offering a singular solution, I do identify certain structural problems and consider corrective measures.

The discussion to follow is organized into eight additional chapters. Chapter 2 outlines the major health planning initiatives associated with each of the periods identified above. Chapter 3 considers the effects of health planning efforts on the structure of the health care system, with particular attention paid to the system of social control associated with each phase. Chapter 4 examines public attitudes as well as scholarly works concerning the health care sector, with special emphasis on the sociology of occupations literature. I focus on this portion of the sociological literature because there is no literature which addresses more specifically the topic of health planning from a sociological perspective. This section argues that the focus of the scholarly work produced during a particular period of time reflects the thinking that prevails in society at that time. Closely related to this argument is the fact that much of the literature on health planning is a product of the spirit of the late 1960s and early 1970s. In effect, I suggest that the larger social context of the time as well as the values that permeated society at that time must be recognized as the backdrop against which the health planning literature evolved. Chapter 5 reviews the literature documenting and evaluating the effectiveness of specific health planning efforts to date. Chapters 6, 7, and 8 report on a number of sociological observations based on twenty months of association with an HSA, where I served in the capacity of participant observer and occasional honorary staff member. The concluding chapter (chapter 9) ties together the ideas presented in the preceding chapters with the aim of assessing the prospects for continuing health planning efforts. The discussion in its entirety should illuminate the underlying thinking, including the assumptions and expectations, behind past health planning endeavors. This, in turn, should lead to a greater appreciation of the sense of disappointment registered by some in response to the realization that many of those expectations were not fulfilled and the satisfaction registered by others who could then hope to see the mechanisms they favored being implemented.

Part I

The History of Health Planning

2

Health Planning Proposals and Programs

The discussion to follow concerns health planning efforts during the twentieth century. Health planning, as indicated in the preceding chapter, is concerned with health care services available to individuals, as opposed to public health measures, which would benefit the community as a whole. In effect, interest in the delivery of health care services to individuals is a twentieth-century phenomenon. Histories of health planning usually begin by discussing the impact produced by the Flexner Report of 1910 (Stebbins and Williams 1972; Hyman 1975).

Included in this outline are proposals, reports, and programs that address the structure of health care delivery systems. The outline employs the four-phase analytical framework discussed in chapter 1. The phases demarcate a shift in thinking regarding health care across three dimensions: first, in the definition of the problem; second, in the mechanisms created to address the problem; and, third, in the preferred locus of social control for implementing the solution. The first two dimensions are the focus of this chapter. The third dimension, locus of social control, is discussed in chapter 3, where the effects of health planning over time are examined.

PHASE I—HEALTH PLANNING VIA PRIVATE SECTOR INITIATIVES

Historical overviews of health planning begin by discussing the Flexner Report of 1910 for several reasons: first, because it marks a major turning point in thinking regarding the value that medical care had to offer to an individual; second, because the changes in the system of medical education that it signaled played a major part in shaping the health care delivery system for decades to come; and, third, there is some suggestion in the literature that health planning would have had a similarly dramatic effect in recent years had health planning structures and processes been designed properly.

While most authors who discuss the events surrounding the Flexner Report would agree that it serves to demarcate the begining of a new era in medical care, not all consider it to be the cause of the new era. Paul Starr convincingly argues that medical education was in the process of changing and the Flexner Report simply accelerated the rate of change (1982; 112–123). He points out that the medical profession initiated its own survey to assess the quality of medical education in 1904. The results were not made public, however, to avoid the intraprofessional unpleasantness which would have certainly resulted, given that many of the medical schools receiving a poor rating were being operated for profit by physicians. The Flexner Report achieved the desired effect without the difficulties that releasing the findings of the profession's internal survey would have created, largely because it was commissioned by a well-known organization outside of medicine, the Carnegie Foundation. Releasing the findings of the report to the public produced an immediate aftermath. The schools receiving poor ratings closed for lack of students, while the highly rated schools became more demanding; they raised entry requirements, expanded the curriculum to include more science and laboratory courses, extended the period of study, and so on.

The Flexner Report is significant for another reason: it reflects the alignment in the thinking of leading physicians and interested laymen regarding the definition of the health care problem and its solution. Representatives of these two sectors agreed that medical science was on the brink of major advances in medical care. This high level of consensus was due, in part, to the growing recognition that medicine was actually achieving more consistent results and, in part, was the result of a steadily increasing level of confidence in any enterprise that could be associated with science. This was the period during which scientific bases were being sought for such varied endeavors as management, child rearing, housekeeping, and so on. The belief that scientific solutions could be found for most if not all of society's ills swept medicine into its tide.

The unprecedented level of confidence in the potential that medical science had to offer, however, was offset by the disappointing realization that a large proportion of physicians currently in practice were unlikely to apply the latest scientific advances because they were not adequately trained to do so. Moreover, it was difficult (then even more so than now) to distinguish between physicians who were competent and those who were not. Thus, it was the concern about the contrast between the variation in quality of medical care currently available as well as the promise that scientific medicine held for the future that gave definition to the health care problem.

That some members of the medical profession were interested in upgrading the quality of medical care is less surprising than the fact that influential persons outside of the profession were becoming concerned about the prevailing quality of medical care. Not only did laymen believe that improved health care was a valuable social good in and of itself, but what is more noteworthy is that they suddenly saw it as an investment promising to bring a high return. These were the wealthy and powerful industrialists of the time who, according to some accounts, thought that improving the health of the workforce would surely lead to improved productivity and, therefore, ultimately result in greater profit (Brown 1979). There is evidence to indicate that this point of view was not seriously challenged for several decades until the Hawthorne study findings were published suggesting that social bonds among workers as well as management's level of interest were more important than working conditions or employee health (Roethlisberger and Dickson 1938). The leading physicians whose training and social status made them an elite, in combination with a small number of the powerful industrialists who were accustomed to having their wishes fulfilled because of their willingness to apply the sheer force of enormous wealth, saw the prevailing problem associated with health care in the same way—poor quality. Furthermore, the two groups were also in agreement about the solution to this problem—improving the quality of medical education. This definition of the problem prevailed until the 1960s. Scientifically grounded medical education, the mechanism that evolved in response to this definition, continued to develop unhampered until then.

Other than the changes in medical education following the release of the Flexner Report, no other major alterations in the health care system initiated by the private sector were implemented during the first half of the twentieth century. However, a number of reports citing various problems and advocating certain changes were published during this period. The Report of the Committee on the Cost of Medical Care, released in 1933, is often cited as an important document, though it did not receive the attention which in retrospect many apparently feel it richly deserved (Falk, Rorem, and Ring 1933; Anderson 1985:94–97). The committee's recommendations are considered noteworthy because the measures advocated are still being discussed—group practice, preventive care, and prepayment. Another major study sponsored by the American Public Health Association and the National Health Council was initiated during this period but not released until 1945. The findings of this study, published as the Emerson Report, are usually described as traditional or conservative, that is, based on a medical approach to illness (Emerson 1945). As a result, this report is considered less interesting than the conclusions reached by the former study. The Ewing Report, issued in 1948, similarly reported on the health of the nation without advocating major changes in the prevailing structure of the system (Ewing 1948). A number of smaller-scale reports appeared during this era as well, aimed at addressing problems posed by particular diseases and sponsored by voluntary organizations associated with the disease, for example, the American Cancer Society and the American Heart Association (Stebbins and Williams 1972).

PHASE II—THE INITIAL STAGE IN PUBLIC SECTOR PLANNING

The next major step in health planning, after the Flexner Report, came in 1946 when the first government-sponsored health planning measure was legislated. With the passage of the Hospital Survey and Construction Act, popularly known as the Hill–Burton Act (PL 79–725), health planning moved out of the private sector and into the public sector.

The intended purpose of the Hill–Burton Act was to shore up the existing network of voluntary hospitals and to stimulate new hospital construction after World War II. Since many hospitals were forced to close during the depression, and few new hospital beds had been added during the war years, the need to encourage hospital renovation and new construction became a high priority during the post-war reconstruction period. The Hill–Burton Act is interesting for an additional reason: it bridges the thinking regarding problems associated with health care arrangements as they were perceived during the first half of the twentieth century with the shift in thinking apparent during the second half of the twentieth century. In fact, the period between 1947 and the mid 1960s constitutes a transition period between the private sector approach to planning prevailing earlier and the public sector approach yet to come.

The main objective of Hill–Burton was to upgrade the quality and quantity of existing facilities, an aim consistent with the priorities existing prior to World War II. The law also emphasized that expansion should be promoted in areas where the need for new beds was greatest. This point of emphasis is now lauded as a significant step forward in thinking regarding health planning. Rural areas and other new population growth areas were thought to be the most likely regions to need added facilities. Public hearings prior to the passage of the act provided the opportunity to introduce the idea that hospital construction should be based on "need." Another innovation of this legislation was that a single agency should be established to oversee the distribution of Hill–Burton funds (McCarthy 1977). Although planning emerged as an important concept during these discussions, little attempt was made to formalize the planning process. This was left to the discretion of the community. Between 1947 and 1974, when Hill–Burton was superseded by the Health Planning and Development Act, however, a series of amendments permitted the government to introduce an increasingly more sophisticated set of formulas to be utilized in determining "need" for additional beds and services.

Hill–Burton was a product of the period immediately after World War II, and it reflected the spirit of the times. This was a reconstructionist era. Americans were eager to get back to peacetime endeavors. Both the pent-up demand for new housing and the consumer goods that go along with an expansion in housing are often credited for producing the economic prosperity of the 1950s. For the most part, this was an era of optimism. However, it was the shift in focus away from international affairs and toward domestic affairs which led to the discovery of major social problems by the end of the decade. The sense that social needs should be examined and addressed was responsible for the creation of a number of government-sponsored blue ribbon committees. In the area of health, the Presidential Commission on the Health Needs of the Nation, created in 1951, produced five volumes of information collectively known as the Magnuson Report (*Building America's Health, 1952–1953*). The volumes contain a detailed report on the then-current status of services, facilities, and manpower. The report also outlined measures to correct deficiencies using federal funds (Stebbins and Williams 1972). Another important study initiated during this period was that of the Commission on Chronic Illness, which was a private sector effort sponsored by the American Medical Association, the American Hospital Association, and the American Public Health Association. Released between 1956 and 1959, the report was the first to bring attention to the health problems faced by older Americans, which the report found to be compounded by their low level of income.

The unwelcome but highly publicized revelations about poverty in the United States made by John Kenneth Galbraith in *The Affluent Society* (1958), by Oscar Lewis in *Five Families* (1959), and by Michael Harrington in *The Other America* (1962) are sometimes credited with playing a crucial role in turning the public's and the government's attention to the existence of poverty and the problems connected to it. The great social awakening taking place at this time resulted in the enthusiasm of the New Frontier approach to social problem solving during the Kennedy presidency and the even more ambitious New Society era during the Johnson years, when the government declared a "war on poverty."

In terms of health care, the perception of the problem had shifted emphasis from concern about improving the quality of health care to the troubling recognition that it was now a highly valued, but scarce, commodity. The new perception of the problem was that some people could not afford to avail themselves of the benefits that a half century of effort devoted to improving the quality of care had produced. The new definition of the problem reflected concern about inequality in the distribution of health care which, it was thought, was due to its scarcity. The solution was obvious—expand the supply of health care services to a level that would respond to the unmet need.

The most significant step taken during this period, in order to assure the availability of health care services to the underserved who were poor and elderly, was the passage of Medicare and Medicaid legislation in 1965 (Social Security Amendments PL 89–97). In retrospect, the major impact on health planning (as opposed to the health of individuals) of these two pieces of legislation can be attributed to the unanticipated extent of the increase in health care costs for which the government was assuming responsibility.

The second major step taken by the government to overcome the newly discovered inequities in access to health care was to increase the supply of health manpower. Several reports were important in focusing attention on the manpower issue: the U.S. Public Health Service estimates of need issued in 1949, the

President's Commission on Health Needs Report of 1953, the National League of Nursing Report of 1957, the Bayne–Jones Report of 1958, the Bane Report of 1959 commissioned by the surgeon general, the Jones Report of 1960, the Task Force on Health Manpower Report that was part of the larger National Commission on Community Health Service Report of 1966, and the report of the National Advisory Commission on Health Manpower issued in 1967. (See Kessel 1970; Fuchs and Kramer 1972, and Reinhardt 1981.)

The first important piece of legislation aimed at resolving the perceived health manpower shortage was the Health Professions Educational Assistance Act (PL 88–129) passed in 1963 and generously amended in 1965 (PL 89–290). A series of legislative efforts with this purpose in mind followed: the Allied Health Professions Personnel Act in 1966 (PL 89–751), the Health Manpower Act in 1968 (PL 90–490), the Health Training Improvement Act in 1970 (PL 91–519), the Comprehensive Health Manpower Training Act in 1971 (PL 92–157), the Nurse Training Act in 1971 (PL 92–158), the Uniformed Services Health Professions Revitalization Act in 1972 (PL 92–426), the Health Revenue Sharing and Nurse Training Act in 1975 (PL 94–94), and the Health Professions Assistance Act in 1976 (PL 94–484). The legislation passed in 1976 signals a shift in the government's approach to the perceived shortage of health care personnel. For the first time the government specified the kind of medical specialists it wanted to support. Funds to medical schools were predicated on setting aside a proportion of places (50% by 1980) for training "primary care physicians" (that is, internists, pediatricians, and specialists in family practice) rather than other types of specialists.

By the latter part of the 1970s some observers were arguing that increasing the supply of health care personnel was creating a greater problem than the one it was intended to resolve because physicians were in a position to create an increased demand for their services. Others insisted that a sufficiently large supply of physicians had not yet been reached to have the desired effect of lowering the cost of care. To date this debate has not been settled (Kessel 1958; Newhouse 1968; Feldstein 1971; Evans 1974; Fuchs 1974 and 1984; Greenberg 1978; Sloan and Feldman 1978; Pauly 1980; Wennberg, Barnes, and Zubkoff 1982).

The third step the government took in response to the health care problem, as it was defined during the 1960s, was to create a structure to allow physicians, as well as the public, to participate in identifying health care needs and in designing plans to address those needs in their own communities. Two pieces of legislation were passsed to accomplish this. First, the Heart Disease, Cancer, and Stroke legislation (PL 89–239), which created the Regional Medical Programs, was enacted in 1965. Second, the Comprehensive Health Planning Program was created by the Public Service Amendments in 1966 (PL 89–749). These two programs were expected to work in conjunction with the Hill–Burton program which had developed guidelines to identify "need" over what was now nearly twenty years of experience.

The Regional Medical Program (RMP) legislation was based on recommendations in the report of the President's Commission on Heart Disease, Cancer, and Stroke (1964). The commission was chaired by Dr. Michael De Bakey, who had recently pioneered open heart surgery in the United States at Baylor University Medical Center. The commission, largely composed of university-based physicians, envisioned establishing regional medical complexes to battle the three leading "killer diseases" via scientific research and technology concentrated in the small number of university-based medical centers where these advances would be implemented. Opposition from the non-academic sector of medicine led to the regional medical program formula emphasizing developing problem solving capability at the level of local institutions. The country was divided into fifty-six program areas based on applications received from regions that largely defined themselves. The organizations originating the proposals varied—thirty-four were university-affiliated, eighteen were non-profit corporations, and four were medical society sponsored (McCarthy, 1977: 357–558). The primary participants were physicians or, as they came to be labeled during this era, providers. The programs also had advisory boards including members of the community who were expected to represent the interests of the public.

The notion that persons other than physicians should be involved in structuring health care delivery arrangements was much more fully developed in the Comprehensive Health Planning legislation (CHP) and the amendments to this law passed the following year (PL 89–749 and PL 90–174). The primary intent of this legislation, also known as the Partnership for Health Program, was to develop plans based on local or regional health needs. The law required the state agency (the "a" agency) to coordinate the overall planning effort. Like the RMP it, too, was expected to rely on an advisory board which was to represent a broad range of interests. The law also created local planning units ("b" agencies) to develop plans for their respective areas based on input from consumer representatives. The law provided for the creation of training programs to prepare the community representatives who had little or no previous experience with the health care system to participate as competent decision makers. Both the "a" and "b" agencies were to include consumers; in fact, the majority (at least 51%) of participants were to be consumers.

PHASE III—THE ADVANCED STAGE IN PUBLIC SECTOR PLANNING

By the early 1970s, the general consensus among observers of the health care system was that a major source of the escalation in costs stemmed from capital expenditures which were not justifiable on the basis of "need." New hospital construction or modernization and the purchase of expensive technological equipment were particularly suspect. (The ranks of interested observers were also swelling because the government was willing to fund research on health care delivery. The volume of literature on this topic expanded rapidly during the period and may have contributed to the speed with which the widely shared belief that capital cost expenditures were responsible for rising health costs was disseminated.) This, in turn, resulted in the amendment to the Social Security Act passed in 1972 (PL 92–603), commonly known as Section 1122. This legislation created a mechanism for reviewing capital expenditures ($100,000 or more) which the states could choose to adopt on a voluntary basis. Disapproval meant that the institution would not receive reimbursement for capital costs usually permitted by the Medicaid, Medicare, and Maternal and Child Health Care programs. When Section 1122 went into effect, fifteen states already had enacted capital expenditure review programs of their own which were being labeled Certificate-of-Need or CON programs. Each state had determined its own guidelines, thresholds, and review procedures (Chayet and Sonnenreich 1978: 5–6).

When it became clear that Section 1122 legislation would not ameliorate the rate of health care cost escalation, many pointed to the flaws in the existing planning laws and argued for more powerful legislation. While the list of deficiencies attributed to the existing planning programs (the RMP and CHP) was a lengthy one, two corrective measures were mentioned most frequently. The consensus was that the planning programs did not achieve their full potential because the consumers were being dominated by the providers and because the laws did not have "teeth." (The literature leading to these conclusions is reviewed in chapter 5.)

The health care problem, as it was conceptualized during the early 1970s, is explicitly stated in the legislation enacted in 1974. The Health Planning and Development Act (PL 93–641) identifies as its purpose the advancement of "equal access to quality health care at a reasonable cost." The definition of the problem as it was perceived during the first half of the century—the need to improve the quality of care—remains; the definition of the problem which followed—the commitment to equalizing access to health care services—is included as well; now a third element—maintaining reasonable costs—is added to the two existing components. In essence, the definition of the problem state by PL 93–641 is a cumulative one. While this view of the problem implies that ambitious solutions were thought to be required, the 1974 legislation was enacted in the spirit of optimism about the effectiveness of the mechanisms provided by the law to address the problem. Herbert Hyman, who authored one of the earliest texts on health planning, captures this sense in the following declaration: "This new law is comprehensive in scope, specific in its language, powerful in its authority, and clear in its intent" (1975: 417).

PL 93–641 specified ten national priorities to guide planning at the state and local level:

1. The provision of primary care services for medically underserved populations, especially those located in rural or economically depressed areas.

2. The development of multi-institutional systems for coordination or consolidation of

institutional health services (including obstetric, pediatric, emergency medical, intensive and coronary care, and radiation therapy services).

3. The development of medical group practices (especially those whose services are appropriately coordinated or integrated with institutional health services), health maintenance organizations, and other organized systems for the provision of health care.

4. The training and increased utilization of physician assistants, especially nurse clinicians.

5. The development of multi-institutional arrangements for the sharing of support services necessary to all health service institutions.

6. The promotion of activities to achieve needed improvements in the quality of health services, including needs identified by the review activities of Professional Standards Review Organizations under part B of title XI of the Social Security Act.

7. The development by health service institutions of the capacity to provide various levels of care (including intensive care, acute general care, and extended care) on a geographically integrated basis.

8. The promotion of activities for the prevention of disease, including studies of nutritional and environmental factors affecting health care services.

9. The adoption of uniform cost accounting, simplified reimbursement, and utilization reporting systems and improved management procedures for health service institutions.

10. The development of effective methods of educating the general public concerning proper personal (including preventive) health care and methods for effective use of available health services. (PL 93–641 January 4, 1975, section 1502)

The law created an extensive network of local agencies, 205 throughout the country, called Health Systems Agencies (HSAs). At the state level two agencies were to review and coordinate various aspects of local agency planning efforts— the State Health Planning and Development Agency (SHPDA) and the Statewide Health Coordinating Council (SHCC). The states could obtain advice from the National Council, mandated to advise the secretary of Health, Education, and Welfare, or from the regional technical centers (there were five) mandated to collect and disseminate information and research.

PL 93–641 supplanted the RMP, CHP, and Hill–Burton program. In doing so the law required that the work of the three programs be assumed by the newly created network of HSAs. It also provided a relatively high level of funding for this assignment (Hyman 1975, 431). The law authorized federal funding at the rate of $.50 per capita plus $.25 per capita (based on population in the HSA planning area) in matching funds.

The two main complaints about previous legislation were addressed as follows: (1) in order to overcome provider dominance, the local and state agencies were mandated to appoint a majority of consumers (over 50% but less than 60%) to their governing boards; and (2) the "teeth" were provided by the CON portion of the law (to equip the agencies with a "bite" as well as a "bark"). Each state was required to pass a CON law by January 1980 to serve as a mechanism for controlling "unnecessary" capital investment expenditures. Hospitals that intended to spend over $150,000, to add ten or more beds, or to introduce certain types of new services were required to submit a proposal to the HSA outlining their plans. The proposed plans were to receive approval at both the local and state agency level. The federal legislation left the issue of penalties for violation of CON decisions to be determined by the states on an individual basis (Lefkowitz 1983, 17). However, serious legal difficulties were implied.

It was intended that a hospital's request for CON approval be considered in the context of plans outlining local needs. The HSAs were expected to develop a five-year plan, the Health Systems Plan (HSP), plus a short-term plan outlining goals for the forthcoming year, the Annual Implementation Plan (AIP). As it turned out, it took more time for the plans to be formalized than expected. This occurred for a number of reasons, including the time required to train new personnel, to collect data on local resources, to develop a health profile of the population in the area, and to decide which needs to address and how to do so. However, the urgency with which cost containment was regarded meant that the CON review process could not await a finished plan. It developed alongside the effort to produce a plan rather than in response to a plan, a point of criticism cited soon after the CON process was instituted.

In fact, the CON portion of the law was receiving criticism even before it was implemented. Institutions were opposed to CON on principle for obvious reasons—they would have to give up a great deal of decision-making autonomy, and they would have to reveal sensitive information regarding the number of procedures being performed, financial resources, special efforts to deal with the poor, and so forth. Thus, the mechanism giving PL 93–641 teeth was also the part of the law most likely to come under attack. Once the CON process was in wide-scale operation, criticism mounted rapidly.

Evaluations of PL 93–641 can be divided into two bodies of literature roughly reflecting the two problems the law was designed to address. First, according to one set of observers, the teeth provided by the law in the form of CON were not working satisfactorily. Second, the problem of provider dominance over consumer representatives still had not been resolved to the satisfaction of other observers. An amendment to PL 93–641 was passed in 1979 (PL 96–79) designed to address both problems. First, the planning agenda was made more specific in order to reinforce the teeth in the law. The 1974 legislation advocated restraint of escalating costs via planning with the aim of avoiding duplication of services and facilities. The 1979 amendments advocated encouraging institutions to share expensive equipment, particularly the single most expensive piece of new equipment in use at the time, the CAT (computerized axial tomography) scanner. The amendments also explicitly stated that cost containment was now a national priority. In fact, the new agenda was to "reduce excess capacity." In order to encourage this plan of action, the 1979 amendments authorized $30, $50, and

$75 million dollars for fiscal years ending in 1980, 1981, and 1982, respectively (HSA working papers n.d.).

Second, the 1979 amendments addressed the problem of provider domination over consumers by changing the basis for selecting consumer representatives. The 1974 legislation required that the consumer representatives "mirror the community." The 1979 legislation, responding to the continuing concern about provider domination of consumers, announced new guidelines for recruiting consumer representatives. They were now to represent specific social, economic, linguistic, racial, and handicapped populations, particular geographic communities within the health service area, and purchasers of health care for collective groups, for example, unions.

The Health Planning and Development Act (PL 93–641) has received a great deal of attention in the form of evaluation research, descriptive commentary, and debate. No one has taken the position, at least not in print, that the law can be considered a total success. While some of the criticism came from persons who hoped their comments would result in changes advancing the regulatory process, there were also those who argued that the entire planning effort should be abandoned because it failed to produce any positive results. These were often the same people who went on to say that a system based on regulatory control was inherently flawed and should be replaced with a market approach based on competition. (See Ginzberg 1982 for review of this debate; for a sharp critique see Thurow 1984).

Even though reports have continued to appear into the 1980s presenting evaluation research results on the successes and failures of PL 93–641, it is clearly no longer the subject of heated debate. Moreover, the general consensus is that the high hopes with which health planning legislation was enacted were not fulfilled. The only remaining point of discussion concerns the merits of continued funding given this negative assessment. To date, the law has not been repealed, but federal funding has been drastically reduced. Furthermore, a number of states have decertified their planning agencies and others are planning to do so. It should also be pointed out that a small number of states have strengthened their planning agencies in recent years.

PHASE IV—HEALTH PLANNING IN THE PRO-COMPETITION ERA

The coming of the 1980s signaled the beginning of the newest phase in health planning. Planning via the public sector was allowed to fade out of existence, to be replaced by the pro-competition approach favored by the Reagan administration and, according to the popular press, favored by industry (Richards 1984). This approach reflects the preferred solution to the revised definition of the problem prevailing at present. Unlike the first three definitions clearly specified during each previous phase, the definition of the problem in the fourth phase is not so clearly labeled. Therefore, I call it "managerial efficiency." The current definition of the problem now consists of the following components: high quality medical care, access for all (this component had been "equal access" previously but is undergoing some revision at present), and cost containment plus efficiency in the delivery of health care.

One of the specific measures adopted by the federal government to encourage efficiency in the delivery of health care comes in the form of the Tax Equity and Financial Responsibility Act of 1982 (PL 97–248) or TEFRA. This legislation empowered the secretary of Health and Human Services to develop a prospective payment system for reimbursement of the hospital portion of health care for Medicare patients. This resulted in the DRG program (diagnostic related groups) enacted as a component of the Social Security Amendments of 1983 (PL 98–21). It is expected that within a three-year phase-in period beginning in October 1983, all of the nation's hospitals would be covered by this program, which is basically a payment system designed to reimburse hospitals on a fixed-fee basis in response to patients' diagnoses. (This is in contrast to the cost-based system which existed previously when the federal government reimbursed hospitals based on the charges they submitted.) Diagnoses have been grouped into 467 DRG categories, plus one "outlier" category for extraordinary cases (468) and two coding problem categories (469 and 470). Teaching hospitals and hospitals in rural areas receive special adjustments to the standard DRG rates.

In order to ensure that providers did not circumvent the system, the government required hospitals to sign agreements by October 1984 with Peer Review Organizations (PROs), which were authorized by the Peer Review Improvement Act as part of the TEFRA Legislation (PL 97–248) of 1982. However, since the guidelines for establishing PROs were delayed, the PRO program began to operate well after it was scheduled to begin ("PRO Rules Criticized . . ." 1983: 2, 10).

Institutions have responded to the dawning of the pro-competition era in health planning by assuming a corporate frame of mind, that is, the same style of thinking and operation that has traditionally been associated with the for-profit sector of industry. Over the space of a very few years, hospitals have formed multi-hospital chains; they have entered into management contracts with hospital management corporations; a number of smaller hospitals have failed; some of these, however, have been returned to service as specialty hospitals under new managment, more often than not operated by a for-profit hospital corporation. Some of the larger medical center hospitals have been spinning off units which charge for their services as independent revenue-producing organizations under a multi-faceted umbrella organization (this is known as "unbundling"). Others have developed new branches offering home health care, emergency care in a free-standing location, plus a variety of other creative approaches to health care delivery (Goldsmith 1981; Starr 1982; Institute of Medicine 1984).

It is noteworthy that the DRG program, the major legislation affecting the health care delivery system to emanate during the current pro-competition era, is, in actuality, heavily dependent on administrative control over reimbursement. Competition occurs in response to a tightly constructed reimbursement structure administered out of Washington, D.C. In a sense, tighter control has been achieved by eliminating the public from the planning structure. The proponents of this approach are claiming, however, that the public has not been eliminated from the planning process but has, instead, been put into a better position to have its demands met via the health marketplace.

CONCLUSION

In sum, four phases in the history of health planning in the United States have been identified. They reflect the fact that perceptions regarding health care problems shifted over time and resulted in four different sets of concerns about health care arrangements. The four definitions of the problem are not, however, distinct. Instead, a new element has been added to the existing definition with each new respective phase. The main problem, during the first half of the twentieth century, was seen as poor quality. During the next stage, roughly the late 1950s to the late 1960s, the problem was identified as unequal access to health care services. This new source of concern did not, however, replace the demand for the highest possible level of health care quality. As of the late 1960s and early 1970s, concern about rising health costs gave the definition of the problem an added dimension. Thus, by the 1970s the problem was defined as a need for high quality care and equal access at a reasonable cost. Finally, with the advent of the 1980s the focus of attention turned to the operation of the health care delivery system. The problems currently being discussed are based on the assessment that the system has been wasteful, duplicative, poorly managed, and lacking in mechanisms which would limit the ability of providers to increase their charges at will. In short, the current definition of the health care problem is that the health care delivery system may be delivering high quality care and making it accessible to a majority of Americans, but it is not doing so at a reasonable cost because there has been no incentive to do so efficiently.

Each of the four phases brought with it a particular set of solutions aimed at addressing the health care problem as it was being defined during each respective period. Accordingly, in phase I, an upgraded system of medical education was expected to raise the quality of medical care. During phase II, a three-pronged approach was employed to increase access: (1) two massive reimbursement programs were created to ensure that the poor and the elderly could afford care; (2) the health manpower supply was increased via an influx of funds to support the expansion of health manpower training; and (3) health planning agencies were created to facilitate both provider and consumer participation in the health planning process. In phase III, the health planning structure was greatly reinforced. Planning agencies were given the power to review and, to some extent, regulate capital expenditure plans proposed by hospitals. The solution, in phase IV, is to encourage institutions to become more efficient by monitoring the cost of caring for patients, specifically Medicare patients. (While the DRG program governs reimbursement for Medicare patients only at present, it is expected to set the pattern for the care of all patients in the near future because private insurance carriers have discovered that institutions have been shifting the costs that government third-party payers would not cover to private third-party payers [Ginsburg and Sloan 1984].)

The changes brought about during each of the four phases contributed to the design of the health care system that has evolved over time. In fact, solutions to earlier problems sometimes produced processes and structures that were themselves thought to require corrective measures during a later period of time. The thinking regarding the locus of control clearly exhibits this pattern. Consider the fact that the profession of medicine was to assume total responsibility for addressing the health problem identified during the Flexner era. This was inherent in the solution provided by the Flexner Report. In phase II, the social programs created during the 1960s shifted the locus of control. Instead of being totally in the hands of the medical profession, the programs were designed with the expectation that the medical profession would be willing to share control on a voluntary basis with members of the public. In other words, the system of control was partially professional and partially administrative.

As of the early 1970s, in phase III, the emergence of a strong reaction against professional control in any form meant that the system of control was to shift from being an arrangement predicated on the voluntary participation of professionals in an administrative control system to a system in which consumer representatives were invested with a majority balance of power over health care professionals. Additionally, the bureaucratic structures created during this era were provided with administrative guidelines and assigned specified regulatory functions. Phase IV constitutes yet another sharp reversal. In the value system characterizing the early 1980s, administrative control is considered to be discredited, and the future development of the health care system is again being returned to the private sector. To be more precise, in the pro-competition era initiated in the 1980s the locus of control has shifted to give the corporate sector of society a greater voice in designing health care delivery arrangements. Thus, the health care system has experienced control via all three of the available social control systems—professional control in phase I, during phase II and III administrative control in two forms, and in phase IV greater control via the marketplace.

To some extent the shifts in social control arrangements can be interpreted as a response to public dissatisfaction with the measures selected to address health sector problems during earlier phases. However, such an explanation would be complete only if the health care system had been operating in isolation, outside the influence of the larger social context in which it exists. In actuality, the shifts in thinking regarding the preferred locus of control apply to a far wider range of social institutions than the health care sector alone. Suffice it to say that the social context of the time played a significant role in the evolution of the health care system in the United States. The larger social context contributed to specifying the health care problem, selecting the solution that best suited the problem, and in assigning the locus of responsibility and control for implementing that solution. While it is not feasible to review the broader historical trends during this time period, I will examine in some detail the growth and development of the health care sector that took place since the beginning of the twentieth century. The following section deals with the effects of the measures that were implemented during each of the four stages in health planning.

3

The Effects of Health Planning over Time

In considering the aftermath of the measures instituted to upgrade the quality of medical care available early in this century, it is important to recognize that the solution selected, and the locus of responsibility for implementing it, stayed in place for more than four decades. By contrast, during the second half of the twentieth century the definition of the problem, the solutions selected to address problems, as well as the locus of control and responsibility for resolving problems have gone through several revisions over the last three decades. The question suggested by this observation is either: Why did the first phase last as long as it did? Or, why are the more recent phases so short-lived? From one perspective, the answer to the question is obvious—the rate at which social changes were occurring was accelerating during these years. From another perspective, the answer is more complicated. It rests on understanding the effects that were produced as a result of the measures adopted to address the problems identified in the first phase of health planning.

The reason for the stability of the first phase can be attributed to the fact that society was reasonably satisfied during that period or, at minimum, not sufficiently dissatisfied to turn its attention from other social concerns to the problem of health care delivery. In order to explicate this line of reasoning, it is necessary to return to the Flexner era.

THE EFFECTS OF THE PURSUIT OF QUALITY

The Flexner Report made explicit to anyone who was interested the standard against which all medical schools were being compared, namely, the Johns Hopkins Medical School. What was significant about the model provided by this institution was its commitment to basic science as an essential prerequisite for training in medicine. The advancement of this approach to medical training was further stimulated by the potential for obtaining generous financial assistance from the Rockefeller and Carnegie Foundations (Brown 1979). The emphasis on scientific medicine produced results in short order. New instruments and techniques began to appear with greater regularity than they had in the past, and improvements in treatment were quick to follow. In fact, medicine was beginning to achieve consistently higher levels of success in applying medical knowledge. This was, of course, the intended outcome.

Another outcome of the focus on scientific advancement, which would prove to be critical to medicine's occupational fortunes in the future, was the fact that an increasing number of physicians affiliated with the leading medical schools were concentrating their efforts on a more narrowly defined set of interests. While groups of physicians with a shared interest in a particular aspect of medical practice had been meeting informally for years, the opportunity to receive training in a specialized area of interest had been a matter of preference and individual enterprise. The focus on improving medical education in general was now also stimulating the emergence of a more organized approach to advanced training in particular areas of practice. Ophthalmologists were the first to develop a specialized program of post-graduate training. The American Academy of Ophthalmology established the first formal specialty program in 1915 when it outlined the scope of training and experience it deemed necessary to declare oneself a qualified specialist; it also instituted an examination and, upon successful completion, awarded a certificate. Thus, the concept of "certified specialist" was born. The otolaryngologists were the next to follow this course in 1924. Between 1930 and 1949 sixteen more specialty certifying boards came into existence. It is important to note that this was not a trend advocated by organized medicine, at least not once the trend toward specialization began to grow at such an unexpectedly rapid pace (Stevens 1971, 198–243). In fact, in 1942, the Advisory Board for Medical Specialties announced that it would not permit additional specialty boards to establish themselves (Stevens 1971, 318–347). However, the process continued as sub-specialty groups proliferated under the auspices of existing boards.

In short, the institutionalization of specialty training began shortly after the release of the Flexner report. This is not to say that medical specialization can be attributed to the report. The report did, however, advocate the advancement of scientifically grounded training, and post-graduate training is simply the logical extension of this emphasis. One way to conceptualize this sequence of events is to view the Flexner Report as the take-off point for a period of unprecedented scientific progress in medicine beginning with the reorganization of medical education but leading eventually to the reorganization of the medical profession itself. At the heart of the matter was the trend toward specialization. While specialization was not an intended outcome of improved medical education, it was, at least initially, considered to be a positive by-product of the emphasis on scientific progress. After all, it did serve as evidence of a rapidly expanding body of scientific knowledge and the existence of a wide range of experts who could apply that knowledge.

The level of confidence in medicine's abilities increased rapidly as a result of the progress it had attained in advancing medical science and the series of steps it took in the effort to assure society that the application of medical knowledge was guided by the highest professional standards. The latter was accomplished through a series of steps sociologists have labeled the "professionalization process." (This process is discussed in greater detail in the following chapter.) It is worth noting, at this point, that the professionalization process was so successful that other occupations sought to emulate the steps taken by medicine. Clearly there was much to be gained in doing so. Not only were generous social rewards, such as high income and prestige, being bestowed on medicine, but professionalization brought with it another major occupational advantage—occupational autonomy. Medicine was entrusted to oversee its own work and to sanction its own members with the support of the state rather than having to accept outside intervention that might prove meddlesome. This is the essence of *professional control*. It is the arrangement that resulted from the social contract between medicine and society and prevailed until the latter half of the 1960s.

At the center of the professionalization process was the main mechanism of control utilized by the profession to advance medical quality—a highly structured and tightly controlled system of medical education. This mechanism was ideal. It matched the purposes of the profession and satisfied the public by reflecting a high level of commitment to professionalism. Far-reaching effects on the practice of medicine could be achieved by manipulating the structure of medical education, without disrupting the lives of the majority of physicians. This meant that the structure of medical education could be extensively altered without encountering opposition from practicing physicians who would not be personally affected. Accordingly, medical education became increasingly more formalized. The institutional framework of the medical educational system served to accommodate the conviction shared by the public that an extensive period of training based on an expanding body of scientific knowledge would produce a cadre of qualified and trustworthy practitioners. The fact that it would take awhile before the effects of changes in the educational system would manifest themselves in practice on a wide scale did not detract from this approach. However, the success of the mechanism rested on the fact that the public did not expect immediate changes during the first half of the twentieth century. Indeed, the public cannot be said to have had any clearly formulated expectations on this matter.

While medical education was becoming highly structured, medical practice remained relatively unstructured, which also fit the prevailing value system in society. Patients were satisfied to have a physician of their own choosing and to develop a personal relationship, usually a long-standing one, without the interference of intermediaries. Physicians were content because they could treat their patients as they saw fit as long as their patients consented to be so treated. Early sociological analyses of medicine indicate that there was considerably more structure in the organization of medical practice than was readily apparent (Hall 1946). However, the network of professional relationships and the bases on which they were constructed were not open to public scrutiny then, nor are they now. Moreover, the public was less inclined to take an interest in such matters, preferring to rely on establishing a better personal relationship with a physician as the best route to quality care. In effect, the structure of medical practice reflected the prevailing social value system which held in high regard freedom of choice and individualism. Clearly, the continued success of this arrangement depended upon the conviction that all physicians were being well trained, so that personal preference rather than client judgment regarding competence could guide the choice of physicians.

With the steady rise in the rate of specialization, the post-graduate medical education system, that is, the residency, superseded the medical school period of training as the arena in which changes in medicine's body of knowledge were introduced. Increasingly, new treatments and techniques were developed by specialists working in university-affiliated medical centers. The organized specialty groups, interested in ensuring that their residents would be the first to learn about the new procedures being developed in their respective areas of medical specialization, took upon themselves the right to approve residency training programs offered by hospitals. Therefore, each specialty group was in a position to determine its own standards and scope of work, that is, its own identity, without any need to take into consideration decisions being made by other specialty groups or by the profession as a whole (DeSantis 1980).

To date, medicine has not found an alternative social control mechanism that is nearly as powerful an instrument for introducing change into the way medicine is practiced. However, introducing changes in medical knowledge and practice to medical students during the medical school period of training rather than during their graduate medical educational training, that is, the residency, had a distinct disadvantage. In the past, changes were introduced informally to the entire cohort of physicians-in-training. As medicine's body of knowledge began to expand more rapidly this arrangement underwent change. Most important was the fact that the proportion of physicians who identified themselves as specialists moved from being a minority to being a majority. By the 1970s medicine had become a loosely organized federation of specialty groups instead of the single, unified profession it had been prior to the acceleration of this trend. The effect of this shift is evidenced by the sharp contrast to an earlier time when the vast majority of physicians shared a uniform identity based on being "physicians and surgeons." In short, in the process of seeking increasingly higher standards of quality, the medical profession underwent a dramatic change in its internal composition, identity, and occupational structure.

From the perspective of society, increasing levels of specialization had been well received in the past because this trend had been viewed as an indicator of the progress that medical science was attaining. However, as the numbers of physicians who declared themselves to be specialists exceeded the number who were willing to engage in general practice, public opinion began to shift. By the end of the 1960s, the observation that it was very difficult to find a family doctor had become a common complaint. People also complained that while physicians may have been treating parts of the body well, the whole person was being overlooked.

The medical profession responded to this criticism in 1971, after a great deal of internal disagreement and difficulty, by establishing a specialty in family practice (Stevens 1971). This response fit medicine's highly successful pattern of accommodating society's demands exhibited in the past. It was employing the medical educational system to introduce an important alteration in the organization of medical practice. Medicine's response, however, was too late and too slow to effect change at the rate being demanded at this point in time. It would take years before the first graduates would be ready to practice and a much longer period of time before a sufficient number of family practitioners would be in practice to cause a noticeable shift in the balance of specialists versus generalists. Society was not content to wait for results as it had in the past. Why society was not willing to wait can best be understood by recalling the larger social context of the time—this was the latter half of the 1960s. Public demands regarding a wide range of social changes were being expressed with a similarly high level of impatience.

THE SHIFT IN PUBLIC ATTITUDE TOWARD MEDICINE

When it came, the reversal in society's stance regarding the benefits of medical specialization was sudden and, as far as the profession was concerned, totally unexpected. Thus, the profession had difficulty absorbing this shift, let alone organizing a suitable response. However, what made the profession's task all the more difficult was the fact that the profession had gone through a metamorphosis that had altered its very nature. This was most apparent in the difficulty medicine was having in attempting to renegotiate its social contract with society. In order to appreciate the impact of the change that specialization had produced in the organization of the profession, one must consider the role played by the American Medical Association (AMA) in the rise of medicine's occupational fortunes.

During the first half of the twentieth century, the AMA consolidated its power, at the peak of which it was able to enroll nearly all practicing physicians in its ranks. Its complex of state and local societies formed a thick communication network with information going up through the system and directives coming down. Although all the members may not have been equally active or even favorably disposed toward the decisions being made at AMA headquarters, the AMA did represent the interests of the majority of its members. This was far easier to do when the majority of its members identified themselves as ''physicians and surgeons,'' that is, general practitioners who combined the practice of medicine with surgery. As specialization began to increase, the split between specialists and general practitioners widened. The specialists divided themselves further by aligning with either medicine or surgery. They could no longer combine both categories of work simultaneously. Those who could not clearly attach themselves to either of these two factions were forced to fend for themselves to protect their area of professional interest. Some, such as pathologists, radiologists, and anesthesiologists, developed institutional alliances with hospitals. More esoteric specialty groups formed coalitions out of necessity rather than mutual interest in one another's work; one of the more extreme examples of such a coalition includes preventive medicine, industrial medicine, aero medicine, and public health (Stevens 1971). With the increase in specialization, members of specialty groups developed interests which did not always coincide with the interests of other members of the profession. In time, specialists were finding that their professional concerns were better met by their specialty organizations (White 1982). As the trend toward specialization increased and more specialists took this stance, the ability of the AMA to affect the professional lives of an increasing number of physicians declined. It was inevitable that this decline in influence would be accompanied by a decline in AMA membership, which began to drop during the 1970s. According to one inside report, it was down to 33% by 1980 (Huffman 1980), and according to the president of the AMA during the following year, it was at about 30% (*New York Times*, June 20, 1984).

Upon reflection there are a number of ironies to be found here. First, it is interesting that the AMA's power was considered to be excessive and dysfunctional (Garceau 1941; Rayack 1967) at exactly the same time that individual physicians were highly regarded by society. It is possible, therefore, that the AMA was performing a "lightning rod" function during this period. In essence, it may have served to absorb the ire of society, so that individual members of the profession were protected. According to Campion (1984), it is Dr. Morris Fishbein who should be credited with the lion's share of responsibility for the negative image attributed to the AMA. Whether it was excessively powerful or not is now moot. What is worth reflecting upon, however, is that physicians were held in high esteem at a time when medicine had far less to offer patients than it does at present (Somers and Somers 1977, 60–75). This is the second irony. Now that medicine has advanced so that it is able to achieve remarkable accomplishments, the individual physicians who perform these feats are thought to be less deserving of the social rewards, especially trust, which were generously bestowed upon physicians in the past. If the decline in the level of confidence society is willing to place in individual physicians parallels the declining influence of the AMA over the members of the medical profession, perhaps the relationship between these two trends merits closer examination. It may just be possible that the AMA's extensive power was functional to the extent that it facilitated delivery on promises made on behalf of the entire medical profession when the AMA engaged in negotiating a social contract with society. Even though the AMA is still generally believed to be very powerful, its power over the majority of practicing physicians is obviously limited to persuasion rather than control, given that 70% of them do not belong to the organization.

The final irony is that in seeking to raise standards of quality in medical practice the small cadre of elite physicians, who were influential in the AMA early in this century, put into motion changes which would ultimately have the effect of weakening its power base. By improving the quality of medical education, the leaders of the profession laid the foundation for specialization, which, in combination with the professionalization strategy, produced an unanticipated but logical outcome. As greater numbers of physicians pursued professionalization on an individual basis, they became more specialized in their work. Membership grew in highly professionalized, clinically oriented specialty organizations, which provided a forum to discuss increasingly more narrow topics of interest. At the same time, the AMA, traditionally more concerned with occupational advancement than scientific matters, lost members. In choosing to join specialty organizations rather than a single, unifying organization, that is, the AMA, physicians were behaving in a highly professional manner. They were also undermining the same organization which had been so effective in negotiating the advantageous social contract medicine enjoyed for many years. The AMA is no longer in a position to fulfill its end of similar social contracts, nor has any other organization appeared to take its place.

THE EFFECTS OF PUBLIC SECTOR HEALTH PLANNING

Phase II in the cycle of health planning efforts was an artifact of the discovery of poverty, problems of aging, inequality in access to health care, and so on. It is important to note that the public attitude toward the medical profession was still highly favorable during this period. Thus, while the programs initiated during this era—Medicare, Medicaid, health manpower expansion, and health planning—may have been opposed by medicine, even vehemently so, they were not enacted with the intention of diminishing medicine's power and control. In fact, it was medicine's response to these programs that partially accounts for the emergence of the negative public sentiment toward medicine that began to take shape at this point in time.

While the medical profession's negative reaction toward the health planning programs enacted during the 1960s is fairly clear, other effects are more difficult to assess for several reasons. For one, so many changes in the health care system were introduced over such a short period of time that the impact of any single program is difficult to isolate. Furthermore, the effects of some governmental efforts would not be apparent as soon as the effects of others. For example, it would take time before the monies allocated to health manpower training would produce any noticeable effects. The health planning legislation was also not expected to produce results immediately. The health planning agencies had to be created first; then community members as well as agency staffs had to become acclimated to their roles; the plans themselves would take time to hammer out; only then could implementation begin to proceed. This is not to say that evaluations regarding the success of planning efforts were not being made, but it would take a number of years before any conclusions based on empirical data would become available. (The evaluation process, its timing, and its impact on the programs being evaluated are discussed in chapter 5.)

That the rising cost of health care would overshadow all other concerns before the salutary effects of programs created to overcome unequal access to health care had time to manifest themselves fully was evident in the earliest comments made by those charged with the implementation of the programs introduced during the 1960s. The extent of the unanticipated increase in health care costs demanded an explanation. The most obvious reason was that the poor, and especially the elderly, had surpassed projected utilization levels. Thus, the blame was initially laid on the people who, it was speculated, were unnecessarily seeking care because it was free. This explanation was short-lived. It was replaced by the assessment that hospitals had adjusted their accounting systems so that they could charge the government for all the new equipment and services they could accommodate (Ehrenreich and Ehrenreich 1970). This assessment gained quick acceptance. Next, the individuals responsible for this agenda had to be identified. The determination was made that physicians were clearly the source of the problem because they were behaving in a fiscally irresponsible manner. (In fact, evidence is just beginning to emerge contradicting the idea that physicians bear primary responsibility for hospital pricing decisions [Bauerschmidt and Jacobs 1985].) It has often been pointed out that physicians have had no incentive to limit their demands for more tests, more equipment, and so forth. In fact, this was the reasoning which led to the enactment of the HMO (Health Maintenance Organization) legislation passed in 1973 (PL 93–222).

The response of the medical profession to the changes being initiated during the 1960s did not make the situation any better. The profession was especially opposed to the Medicare and Medicaid programs (Colombotos 1969; Ehrenreich and Ehrenreich 1970). This reaction made medicine appear callous and uncaring about the needs of the poor and elderly. The medical profession was thought to be acting strictly in a self-interested manner, which went against the groundswell of popular feeling. There was little public recognition that this may have been less a case of inadequate humanitarian concern and more a matter of resisting the shift from a system of *professional control* over the health care structure to the introduction of *administrative controls*, even if these were relatively unrestrictive at this stage. Why physicians would fight the imposition of administrative controls of any sort should not be difficult to understand. Why they were so aggressive about it becomes apparent when one considers the extent of the loss of occupational autonomy involved. Consider the fact that discussions regarding expansion of particular hospital services, the addition of new beds, and the purchase of new equipment were going to be reviewed by outsiders. Such decisions previously had always been made behind closed doors. Hospital board members were involved, of course, but discussions with board members generally proceeded in the congenial atmosphere of a private club over drinks and lunch. In this new atmosphere, physicians were being told they would have to present data publicly on the number of procedures their service performed, how their hospital planned to fund the project, and why they thought they needed to expand. All this would take place before uninformed members of the public, colleagues (possibly unfriendly ones) from neighboring institutions, other hospital employees, and so on. Physicians were being asked to accept the shift from a system over which they had total control for many years to sudden intervention at many levels. The fact that the programs were intended to be supportive rather than punitive did not make them any more palatable. From the perspective of the public, however, the fact that the intent was to be supportive of medicine's efforts made its seemingly extreme reaction all the more difficult to comprehend.

The medical profession's resistance to programs which would permit needy people to obtain health care, followed by reports that once the Medicaid and Medicare programs were in effect the health care system was using the programs to benefit itself, ultimately fueled the shift in public attitude toward medicine (Stevens 1971, 485). The AMA opposed programs which would provide care for anyone who was not truly needy (which would have to be proven via a means test). This reaction, in addition to the fact that people claimed they could no longer find a family physician but had to go from one specialist to another for each separate problem (in effect, from one stranger to another), exacerbated the negative public reaction, the fact that the same people rushed to seek out the "best specialist" when something really serious was perceived to be wrong not withstanding. This is the scenario evolving during the same era that the social turmoil beginning in the 1960s was in full swing. It was at this point that society's confidence in medicine as a social institution also began its decline.

Medicine for its part attempted to respond to the new set of social demands by using familiar mechanisms proven successful in the past. It continued to focus its energies on technological progress, renewed its efforts to improve the quality of medical education, and emphasized its successes on the medical research front. Support for advancing medicine's body of knowledge seemed to be getting a positive response in the form of RMP funding for advancing its technological capacities during the late 1960s. Not knowing how to conquer the leading "killer diseases," which was one of the new publicly announced demands confronting medicine, physicians directed their efforts toward saving the lives of those who were in a critical stage of illness. Intensive care technology, which was greatly advanced during this period (Russell 1979), seemed to generate a positive social response for a time.

The measures taken by medicine during this period, however, did not prove to be enough. Not only did the public continue to withdraw its confidence from medicine, but malpractice suits were rising, reaching an unprecedented peak by 1974 (Stroman 1979). The courts were slowly beginning to erode certain professional prerogatives; for example, the prohibition against advertising was being reconsidered. On another front, in a landmark case (*Darling v. Charleston Community Hospital*), a hospital was penalized because it did not take responsibility for evaluating the qualifications of physicians on its staff, specifically the staff physician who was serving on rotation in the emergency room. This resulted in the imposition of administrative controls over physicians at the local hospital level. Another stinging blow came from Ralph Nader's forces, who publicly challenged medicine's performance in monitoring its membership (Keelty et al. 1970). The document produced by this group, entitled *One Life—One Physician*, is credited by some for pressuring the government into legislating a formally organized monitoring structure (Sheldon 1975,44–62). The 1972 PSRO (Professional Standards Review Organization) legislation (PL 92–603) was passed around this time.

With the beginning of the 1970s, it was clear that there would be no turning the tide of sentiment demanding greater administrative control over the health care structure in general and the medical profession in particular. In fact, there was a growing sense that the *voluntary administrative control* arrangements inaugurated during the latter half of the 1960s, in the form of the RMP and CHP, had permitted the providers to dominate planning efforts. This was the climate spawning the third stage of health planning—*administrative control* based on *regulation*.

THE LEGACY OF PUBLIC SECTOR HEALTH PLANNING

Public sector health planning efforts, together with other public programs aimed at improving health care arrangements, launched during the 1960s did not produce the effects that were anticipated. This resulted in an even greater level of commitment to a public sector or *administrative control* approach to resolving the problems associated with health care delivery. In short, the public sector health planning programs of the 1970s were inaugurated in reaction to the experience of the 1960s. This includes the experience of attempting to effect specific changes in the health care delivery system, experience in dealing with the resistance of the medical profession to the social agenda of this period, and, perhaps even more important, the overall experience of living through the period of social turmoil of the late 1960s. The legislation of the 1970s was purposeful in withdrawing a large share of medicine's social mandate and placing it in the hands of the public. This was accomplished by according majority status to "consumer representatives" in the health planning structure in order to ensure that "providers" would not be in a position to play the dominant role in directing the future development of the health care system.

Whether one concludes that the mechanisms associated with *administrative control* succeeded or not depends to a large extent on one's disposition toward the *market system of control*, which has edged out the administrative controls implemented during the second and third health planning phases. Before considering the arguments on the merits of these systems or the literature addressing the successes and failures of health planning during the period of public sector planning, one must consider first the evidence documenting the shift in attitude toward the health care system in general and medicine in particular over time. The following chapter discusses the relationship between the locus of social control and shifts in public attitude regarding the health care system.

4

The Rise and Decline of Professional Control

The shift in public attitude toward the medical profession which occurred toward the end of the 1960s is a significant turning point because it constitutes the watershed in thinking regarding the preferred locus of control over the health care system. The preceding chapter argued that the medical profession's fortunes soared during the first half of the twentieth century largely because its occupational outlook fit so well the prevailing value system. The medical profession was given a great deal of autonomy to conduct its affairs and, more importantly for purposes of this discussion, to assume responsibility for the direction in which the health care system would evolve. This was an era when professionalism grounded in scientific expertise was thought to be the ideal form of institutional leadership and control. In other words, an examination of the evolution of the medical profession must take into consideration the larger social context prevailing at that time. Although this may be obvious, it has not prevented many observers of the medical profession from treating it as if it existed in isolation from major events and ideas that govern the society in which the medical care system exists.

The following discussion addresses, first, the timing of the change in public attitude during the late 1960s and early 1970s toward the medical profession and, second, factors that have been mentioned to explain this shift. However, the principal idea conveyed in this chapter concerns the relationship between scholarly analyses and prevailing social thought. (The meaning attached to the latter concept encompasses public attitudes and popular interpretations of current events.) Basically, I contend that the thinking expressed in scholarly works attracts acclaim from members of the scholarly community because it closely approximates more general public sentiments. Accordingly, the highly acclaimed scholarly analyses produced during earlier periods of time must be viewed as accurate reflections of their respective periods in time. In order to develop the implications that follow from these assessments in greater detail, I consulted the literature on occupations and professions for illustrative purposes. This body of literature also provides the backdrop for understanding the dramatic shift in thinking regarding the locus of social control that occurred during the late 1960s. This chapter concludes by pointing out that the health planning literature should be viewed from a similar perspective—as a reflection of the thinking that prevailed in society at the time that this body of literature was produced.

THE TURNING POINT IN PUBLIC SATISFACTION

In examining the evidence documenting the shift in attitudes regarding the organization and control of health care delivery arrangements, one should note that the surveys addressing the public's attitudes about the health care system did not begin until the 1970s. Prior to this time, the focus of public interest was on the profession of medicine rather than health care. Since the medical profession was primarily responsible for overseeing the growth and development of the health care system prior to the late 1960s, evidence of society's reactions to medicine prior to this time will be treated as a proxy measure for society's reaction to prevailing health care arrangements. However, it is important to remember that medicine in this context does not refer to organized medicine, a label generally identified with the AMA. There is little evidence to suggest that the AMA has ever been highly regarded by the public, with the possible exception of the Flexner era, when it became actively involved in the effort to upgrade the quality of medical education.

The shift in public sentiment toward the medical profession has not received as much attention as we might expect given its significance. It came at a time when medicine was at the pinnacle of occupational success. Consider the evidence. First, in terms of income, the medical profession seems to have become the top-paying occupation during the early 1940s (see Table 1). According to the Bureau of Labor Statistics (1982), it slipped to sixth place between the 1970 and 1980 census. The 1983 Bureau of Labor Statistics data find physicians in seventeenth place (1985). This is due, in large part, to the fact that individuals who are incorporated are not included in the survey, and over the last decade many physicians took this step. By contrast, the *Medical Economics* statistics indicate that physicians' incomes have risen significantly in the recent years. The point I wish to stress is that physicians' incomes rose more rapidly than those of other occupational groups just after World War II at about the time that the value of what medicine had to offer was gaining wide recognition.

Second, when the results of the first North–Hatt survey on prestige were published in 1947, medicine was rated second, out of ninety occupations, after supreme court justices. The second time the survey was conducted in 1963 medicine's rank remained the same (see Table 2). (Unfortunately, neither this survey nor a similiar survey was conducted after this time.) Third, answers to

Table 1
Occupational Earnings by Selected Occupation

	Physicians[a]	Physicians[b]	Lawyers[b]	Dentists[b]	Engineers[c]
1929[1]	$ 5,806[6]	$ 5,224	$ 5,534	$ 4,267	$ 3,468
1940[1]	4,470[7]	4,507	4,507	3,314	3,324
1945[1]	8,688[8]	10,975	6,861	6,922	4,908
1950[1]	15,262 mean[9] 13,150 median[9]	12,324	8,349	7,436	6,216
1960[2]	22,100[10]	24,300	---	14,747	---
1969[3]	40,550[11]	25,000+	18,749	21,687	14,888
1981[4]	83,700[12]	29,172	29,848	---	31,940
1983[5]	94,580[13]	26,208	32,344	---	32,456

[a]Data from Medical Economics Company, Inc., Oradell, N.J.; 1928 and 1939 figures are based on the "average" or mean net income; 1951 figures report a mean and median figure; in all years after 1951 the figure reported is the median; see references 6 through 13 for specific citations.

[b]Bureau of the Census and Bureau of Labor Statistics; see references 1 through 5 for specific citations.

[c]David Blank and George Stigler, The Demand and Supply of Scientific Personnel (New York, 1957), National Bureau of Economic Research, pp. 114, 116. 1940 figure reflects data for 1939; 1945 figure reflects data for 1946; 1950 figure reflects data for 1953; 1969, 1981, 1983 data correspond to references 3, 4, and 5, respectively; however, it must be noted that these data are for aerospace engineers since this is the subdivision of engineers found first in the listing of engineering salaries.

[1]Bureau of the Census, Historical Statistics of the United States, Colonial Times to 1970, Part 1, Bicentennial ed., 1976, pp. 175-176 (average annual net income).

[2]Figures for dentists for 1961; figures for physicians for 1962; from Bureau of the Census, 1976.

[3]Dixie Somers, "Occupational Rankings for Men and Women by Earnings," Monthly Labor Review 97 (August 1974): 35. (Data refer to median annual earnings for males.)

[4]Bureau of Labor Statistics, "1981 Weekly Earnings of Men and Women Compared in 100 Occupations," News release (March 7, 1982), USDL 82-86.

[5]Earl Mellor, "Weekly Earnings in 1983: A Look at More than 200 Occupations," Monthly Labor Review 108 (January 1985): 54-59.

[6]William Alan Richardson, "Our Post-Depression Incomes," Medical Economics (April 1934): 12-14, 77-81. (Data for 1928)

[7]"Physicians' Incomes," Medical Economics (September 1940): 38-48. (Data for 1939)

[8]"Physicians' Economic Status," Medical Economics (November 1944): 48-49. (Data for 1943)

[9]"Your Economic Weather Vane," Medical Economics (December 1952): 71-87, 121-125. (Data for 1951)

[10]"How Your Earnings Compare," Medical Economics (October 24, 1960): 38-47. (Data for 1959)

[11]Arthur Owens, "Inflation Closes in on Physicians' Earnings," Medical Economics (December 21, 1970): 63-71. (Data for 1969)

[12]Ibid., "How's Inflation Treating You?" Medical Economics (September 28, 1981): 173-185. (Data for 1980)

[13]Ibid., "Are You Still Losing Out to Inflation?" Medical Economics (November 1944): 48-49. (Data for 1983)

Table 2
Occupational Prestige Rankings

Occupation	1947 Ranking[1]	1963 Ranking[2]
U.S. Supreme Court Justice	1.0	1.0
Physician	2.0	2.0
State Governor	2.0	5.5
Cabinet Member in Federal Government	4.0	8.0
Diplomat in the U.S. Foreign Service	4.0	11.0
Mayor of a Large City	6.0	17.5
College Professor	7.0	8.0
Scientist	7.0	3.5
U.S. Representative in Congress	7.0	8.0
Banker	10.0	24.5
Nuclear Physicist	18.0	3.5
Government Scientist	10.5	5.5
Chemist	18.0	11.0
Lawyer	18.0	11.0

[1]National Opinion on Occupations, final report, NORC, University of Denver, April 22, 1947.

[2]Robert Hodge, Paul Siegel, and Peter Rossi, "Occupational Prestige in the United States: 1925-1963," NORC draft of survey no. 466, 1964.

the following Gallup survey question provide added evidence of the high regard the public has had for the medical profession: "Suppose a young man asked you about taking up a profession, which would you recommend?"

Fourth, the National Opinions Research Center and Harris surveys on confidence in various social institutions provide the best evidence of the position that medicine as a social institution had attained by the mid 1960s. The survey question both have asked is: "I am going to name some institutions in this country. As far as the *people running* (emphasis in original) these institutions are concerned, would you say you have a great deal of confidence, only some confidence, or hardly any confidence at all in them?" The range of answers includes: a great deal, only some, hardly any, don't know and no answer. The percentage of the total answering "a great deal" is reported in Table 4.

Table 4 also makes clear the fact that the public was beginning to lose confidence in medicine by the early 1970s; however, this fact must be viewed in the larger context. In this light, it is apparent that medicine suffered far less than other social institutions included in the survey on confidence. Thus, the shift in attitude toward medicine cannot be treated as an isolated phenomenon. Medicine was being swept along in the turmoil of social change. Indeed, the fact that it retained more public confidence during the late 1960s and early 1970s than many other social institutions deserves greater recognition than it has received to date (Blendon and Altman 1984).

A variety of explanations has been proposed in an attempt to understand this period of social turmoil; none has proven to be wholly satisfying. Therefore, I

Table 3

Careers Recommended to Young Men (reported as a percentage)

Career	1953[1]	1962[2]	1973[3]
Doctor	29%	23%	28%
Engineer-Builder	20	18	13
Business Executive	7	5	10
Clergyman	7	8	7
Lawyer	6	6	14
Dentist	6	4	7
Professor-Teacher	5	12	10
Government Career	3	7	5
Veterinarian	3	–	–
Banker	2	2	2
Other	4	4	4
None, I don't know	8	11	

[1] George Gallup, The Gallup Poll, Public Opinion, 1935-1971 (New York: Random House, 1972), p. 1152.

[2] Ibid., p. 1779.

[3] George Gallup, The Gallup Poll, Public Opinion, 1972-1977 (Wilmington, Del.: Scholarly Resources, Inc., 1978), p. 216.

offer an explanation requiring that we recognize the highly charged feelings that American society has had about science at least since the turn of the century if not before. Recalling the Flexner era, science was invested with great expectations. It was harnessed in a number of arenas so that scientific discoveries could be turned into practical, technological by-products. This arrangement and the pace at which scientific progress was moving was apparently considered to be satisfactory until the Soviet Union launched *Sputnik* in 1957. At that point, Americans marshaled extensive forces to cope with this event, which was received as a devastating blow to American pride. The immediate effect was a tremendous emphasis on science education in order to produce more and better scientific experts. It did not take long before society determined that an overcorrection had occurred. Well-known individuals began to voice concerns about the dangers inherent in permitting technologically sophisticated experts to influence important decision-making processes. General Eisenhower shocked America with the warning that a military–industrial complex had come into existence. John Kenneth Galbraith identified the locus of power in the corporation as the technostructure (1967). A surge of interest in topics such as scientific paradigms (Kuhn 1970), the scientific community (Crane 1972), and little science versus big science (De Solla Price 1963) captured the attention of social scientists during this period as well. If the experts were suddenly being viewed with suspicion, "the people" were gaining confidence in their own assessments bolstered by the growth in numbers of people opposed to the Vietnam war. The public was vindicated. About the time that the war was over and society was determined

Table 4

Confidence in Social Institutions Survey

1966 Ranking	Institution	1966[1]	1967[1]	1970[1]	1973[2]	1975[3]	1978[3]	1980[3]	1982[3]	1983[3]	1984[3]	1984 Ranking
1	Medicine	72	61	61	54	50	46	52	45	51	50	1
2	Banks/Financial	67	54	36	—	32	33	32	28	24	31	5
3	Military	62	56	27	32	35	29	28	31	29	36	3
4	Education	61	56	37	37	31	28	30	33	29	28	8
5	Scientific Community	56	45	32	37	38	31	41	32	41	44	2
6	Major Companies	55	47	27	29	19	22	27	23	24	30	7
7	Supreme Court	50	40	23	31	31	28	25	30	28	33	4
8	Congress	42	41	19	23	13	13	9	13	10	12	12
9	Organized Religion	41	40	27	35	24	31	35	32	28	31	5
10	Executive Branch	41	37	23	29	13	12	12	19	13	18	9
11	Press	29	27	18	23	24	20	22	18	13	17	10
12	Television	25	20	22	18	18	14	16	14	12	13	11
13	Organized Labor	22	20	14	15	10	11	15	12	8	8	13

[1] Tom Smith, "Can We Have Confidence in Confidence? Revisited", Denis Johnston (ed.), Measurement of Subjective Phenomena (Washington, D.C.: U.S. Bureau of the Census, 1981), pp. 119-189.

[2] General Social Surveys, 1972-1982: Cumulative Codebook (July 1982), NORC, pp. 111-114.

[3] General Social Surveys, 1972-1984: Cumulative Codebook (July 1984), NORC, pp. 152-155.

to return to peacetime affairs, there was renewed reason to distrust experts in yet another arena. Watergate provided convincing evidence that political experts also did not deserve our trust.

This is the developing scenario to which a second reason for the shift in attitude toward medicine can be attributed. While scientific progress was highly valued in the past, it was now becoming overwhelming. One of the central themes inherent in the American value system was, and is, that success depended on one's wit and personal effort. If there is too much technical information for any one person to master, it undermines the decision-making independence of the individual. Furthermore, one becomes dependent on experts who do not take the time to explain things so that the matter can be easily understood. This point of frustration is closely related to the widespread notion that experts in various fields, medicine in particular, were hoarding knowledge to maintain their respective positions of power and that when they did explain things in easily understandable terms, they were being condescending. Even worse, the experts were becoming increasingly more prone to disagreeing with one another. According to the popular wisdom this can only be because somebody is advocating an option from which he stands to profit. Worst of all, however, the experts remained sufficiently loyal to one another to prevent them from revealing whose solution was the unnecessary but profitable one. This is in sharp contrast to the relatively recent past when one could take care of most problems oneself. When one did seek professional help, there was usually a single, clearly advisable, relatively uncomplicated solution; moreover, the professional/expert was likely to be a member of the community who was well known and trusted. The new breed of experts coming on the scene was just the opposite.

This generalized set of explanations paralleled exactly the conventional wisdom which evolved to explain the fact that an increasing number of physicians were identifying themselves as experts or specialists rather than general practitioners. The belief that physicians are primarily motivated by the potential of greater economic gain achieved widespread acceptance during this era. This perspective also facilitated the linking of the main points of dissatisfaction with regard to the medical profession that emerged during the late 1960s, namely, high cost and inadequate humanitarian concern about patients. While financial gain is no doubt an important factor in explaining the rise of medical specialization, accepting this as a total explanation is simplistic. I contend that the trend toward specialization has been central to the growth of the public dissatisfaction with medicine and can be better understood by using a broader explanatory framework than one that depends on an assessment made about the psycho-social motivational systems of a large number of individuals, that is, doctors. We must look more closely at the value system of the society in which a formal system of specialization took hold. To begin with, there was society's demand, at least on the part of certain influential representatives of that society, that medicine be grounded in science, an aim greatly encouraged by vast sums of money. Additional support for choosing to specialize can be attributed to the symbolic meanings as well as financial advantages accrued to specialists. It is not only that specialists would be paid more than generalists for performing identical services, but that they would also be recognized as better qualified. To illustrate, specialists have long been called upon to testify as expert witnesses in court procedures; during World War II, they were given a higher rank, more pay, and more privileges, including being assigned to field hospitals while general practitioners were sent to the front (Stevens 1971); and, in the end, they flourished because patients were eager to seek them out and pay a premium fee for care by a recognized expert.

In essence, a number of extrinsic rewards other than financial gain contributed to the trend toward specialization. Certain intrinsic rewards might also be mentioned. Even apart from the inner reward that comes from "doing good," there is the satisfaction produced by the sense of mastery over one area of medicine that being a generalist may not provide. The reverse of this is also worth considering, that is, a sense of insecurity about one's knowledge of the entire field of medical practice can be avoided by narrowing one's focus (Becker 1961) or (to use a concept borrowed from a discussion on a different topic) by limiting the "scope of one's liability" (Janowitz 1952). In sum, there is no question that society advocated medical specialization during the first half of the century, but that by the 1960s society was dissatified for a number of reasons with the extent to which medicine had become specialized. More importantly, the attribution of financial motivation for the rise in specialization has been applied retrospectively in the wake of the shift in public attitude toward medicine.

THE SOCIOLOGY OF OCCUPATIONS AND PROFESSIONS

The emergence of retrospective and revisionist interpretations is not an exclusive property of the popular wisdom realm of explanations. In fact, at the heart of the point to be made in this discussion is the observation that major shifts in perspective found in scholarly analyses are accompanied by an effort to discredit earlier interpretations in order to provide greater support for the newly revised interpretation. To illustrate, consider the body of literature classified as the sociology of occupations and professions; more recently, this literature also has been labeled the sociology of work (see Smigel 1954 and 1963 for a discussion of sociological interest in this topic). This literature is the focal point because it is the only body of literature in sociology which has had a continuous tradition of interest in the medical profession and the social circumstances in which it conducts its work. What I propose to do at this point is to treat the body of sociological literature on occupations and professions itself as a data source, the premise being that sociological writing on the professions constitutes an historically accurate picture of the thinking that prevailed over time not only among sociologists but in society at large.

One question that fascinated sociologists interested in work earlier in this century was: What makes medicine different from other occupations? (Carr-

Saunders 1933; Greenwood 1957; Goode 1960; Barber 1963; Moore 1970). Another version of this question puts the underlying perspective into better focus: What are the characteristics of medicine that make it more successful than other occupations? In short: What are the reasons that other occupations are in an inferior position to that occupied by medicine? It was necessary to begin by specifying occupations that were successful and those that were not. This was done on a continuum starting with old, established professions through to the new professions, the semi-professions, the would-be professions and finally the marginal professions (Reiss 1955). The fact that such typologies inspired a good deal of interest among sociologists indicates that the potential answer was thought to be a valuable one (Etzioni 1969). There was also a considerable amount of attention paid to the steps that medicine pursued to attain its enviable occupational position. Many occupations, undoubtedly unaware of Caplow's (1954), Wilensky's (1964) and Gross' (1958) observations, used similar tactics to upgrade their standing. They changed their names (from mortician to funeral director, from janitor to maintenance engineer, from beautician to cosmetologist, and so on); formed professional associations; launched journals; pressed to upgrade educational requirements; and instituted licensure examinations. The sociologists, for their part, were attempting to identify ingredients of a socially valued pattern of action occupational groups were eager to employ in pursuit of the rewards that society was obviously willing to bestow on those who successfully completed the professionalization process.

Some sociologists took a distinctly neutral stance toward the process of occupational development. They neither advocated the professionalization process nor did they criticize those who did. Everett Hughes and many of the sociologists he influenced during their graduate school years fall into this category (Lortie 1958; Becker 1961; Bucher 1962; see Dingwall 1983 for discussion of Hughes' influence). It was Hughes who observed that medicine had attained an exclusive "license" and broad social "mandate" over medical work (1958). He also pointed out that even as society awarded medicine its highly privileged position, medicine continually pressed for more (Ritzer 1977, 41–67; Starr 1982).

Talcott Parsons was the primary proponent of the school of thought which saw the relationship between medicine and society as a highly functional one (1951). According to Parsons there were good reasons to reward the medical profession extremely well. He pointed to the weighty responsibilities that medicine was willing to assume; of special significance was its role in controlling malingering. Parsons argued further that the elevated status accorded to physicians was essential to ensure a high level of respect, which would lead to proper cooperation from patients. He concluded that the arrangement was functional—physicians performed crucial services for society under a stringent set of conditions for which they deserved to be well rewarded.

Such assessments may appear naive at this point in time. However, that is not the same thing as saying the assessments were wrong for the time during which they were made. In support of this point, I might note that there is little variation in the perspective that sociologists maintained in studying the professions, medicine in particular, prior to the 1970s. This may be due to the existence of a widely shared, among sociologists and the general public alike, set of values that held professionalism and expert knowledge in high regard.

A similar statement can be made about the literature on the professions after 1970; public opinion and sociological thinking moved concurrently toward a new conclusion at this time. Without doubt Eliot Freidson's two books served to inaugurate the new era in sociological thinking with regard to the medical profession (1970 and 1970). While Parsons had found the social arrangement that evolved between medicine and society to be functional, Freidson argued that this relationship was dysfunctional and took the position that medicine's power had become excessive. However, Freidson also stated that colleague-centered referral networks delivered medical care that was superior to the care that was likely to be forthcoming from client-centered referral networks. This was because a professional system of control was better suited for judging the quality of medical treatment than was a control system that was primarily responsive to consumer satisfaction. If professional control was functional at this level, in what sense was it dysfunctional? Freidson identified the dysfunctional aspect as "professional dominance" (1970). The focus of his discussion is directed at the attitude and behavior of physicians on a one-to-one basis toward those around them, that is, patients and the members of other health occupations. Freidson's observations were primarily concerned with the domineering behavior exhibited by some physicians at the level of interpersonal interaction (Freidson 1985).

Freidson's work was very well received by sociologists as well as health system analysts from other disciplines. In fact, the meaning attached to the concept of "professional dominance" was used so frequently that it evolved to encompass a far more comprehensive meaning than the one originally assigned by him. The concept became the foundation for proposals suggesting that medicine's license and mandate should be severely restricted (Daniels 1973; Halmos 1973; Haug 1973). The sociologists who advocated this line of thinking can be said to belong to what is known as the conflict school of thought. Conflict theorists espouse the belief that physicians achieved their socially advantageous position by using power tactics, that is, overcoming competitors, maintaining exclusionary controls over medical knowledge, and using political machinery to legitimate their efforts.

In short, the timing of the shift in perspective found in sociological thought parallels the shift in public opinion. When public opinion regarding medicine was favorable, the earlier sociological literature, written from a functionalist point of view, focused on the qualities possessed by medicine which were responsible for its occupational success. When public opinion shifted, so did the focus of the sociological literature concerned with occupations and professions. In sum, the conflict theory perspective gained ascendancy at this particular time because it fit the prevailing value system of the time.

This observation may or may not be viewed as provocative. My interpretation of the consequences of the relationship between public opinion and sociological writings may have this effect, however when one considers that sociology as a discipline overreacted to the conflict theory critique. Sociologists accepted too readily the notion that earlier sociological analyses of the professions were naive and perhaps even somewhat embarrassing. The effort to discredit these earlier works should be reconsidered. In fact, it would be more accurate to conclude that the sociological analyses presented by the functionalists as well as those of the conflict theorists constitute an accurate representation of the thinking of their time. The functionalists reflected the prevailing perspective of their time, which was a steadily rising regard for medicine as a profession. The conflict theorists captured the newly emerging perspective at the same time that the medical profession's occupational position entered into a declining phase. Thus, neither perspective is wrong; the period of time involved is simply different. This point would be less significant if it were not for the fact that sociologists virtually abandoned the study of occupations altogether in response to the revisionist attack on earlier work launched by the conflict theorists. Fortunately, there are signs that this effect is wearing off (Betz and O'Connell 1983; DeSantis 1983; Dingwall and Lewis 1983).

PUBLIC OPINION AND SOCIOLOGICAL THINKING IN THE 1980s

The degree of interest and widespread acclaim accorded to Paul Starr's (1982) book on the medical profession indicates that another shift in attitude toward medicine is taking place. Starr distances himself from the conflict theory interpretation of medicine's rise and subsequent decline in occupational fortunes. He maintains that the medical profession had been pursuing the same tactics throughout its history with little visible success. He points out that medicine achieved a positive social reaction to its demands in the twentieth century only because society was prepared to accord medicine the recognition and rewards it had sought all along. His stance becomes even more explicit when he suggests that the self-serving antics of the medical profession are now beginning to appear petty and fumbling in contrast to the agenda of the corporate health industry currently taking shape.

Accepting the assessment that a shift in sociological thinking regarding medicine is now taking place, my interpretation of the relationship between sociological writings and public opinion in the past should predict to a similar trend in the future. Public opinion should be moving in the same direction as sociological assessment. I would argue that it is, even if it is difficult to support this observation more conclusively. It seems that recent public opinion polls regarding medicine and/or the health care sector have resulted in a complex set of answers, causing a considerable amount of consternation to anyone interested in analyzing them (Blendon and Altman 1984; Iglehart 1984). For one, the polls consistently reveal that the public is willing to pay more for health care services. This is difficult to reconcile with the message coming from the public media or the response being registered in Washington, D.C. Furthermore, the fact that a majority of people believes that the health care system is in a state of crisis, and, at the same time, that a majority is satisfied with its own care is causing attitude survey analysts to interpret their findings very cautiously (Andersen, Fleming, and Champney 1982).

According to one of the most recent and comprehensive interpretations, the polls indicate the existence of a national schizophrenia but not an inexplicable one (Blendon and Altman, 1984, 613–616). Blendon and Altman interpret the surveys as follows: (1) the rising cost of care is the number one problem in health care; it is not, however, thought to be the most important problem facing the nation now; (2) most Americans are troubled by the high cost of health care but not by the share of the GNP devoted to health care; (3) most Americans believe that the current structure of the health care system should be reorganized, but they are not willing to alter their own health-seeking patterns of behavior; (4) most people do not consider themselves responsible for rising health care costs, therefore, they support only those cost-containment measures that leave their own health care arrangements in tact; (5) the views of physicians regarding proposals to change the system carry more weight than the opinions of those attempting to introduce changes. In the end, the authors conclude that little change is likely because of the lack of consensus regarding possible solutions.

THE HEALTH PLANNING LITERATURE

A noteworthy gap in the health care literature is the lack of any information on how or where consumers/patients obtain information about personal health matters or about the health care system as a whole, that is, how good the quality of care is, what it costs, who makes decisions about the system and so forth. Although the public has opinions on these matters, we know little about the source of the information on which these opinions are based. It is likely that public opinion is based on sophisticated information produced by researchers and translated for public consumption by reporters via the press, radio, and television. A great deal of information is issued by spokesmen who represent interested institutions (for example, government agencies, the AMA, the American Hospital Association, medical specialty societies, voluntary associations, insurance carriers, labor representatives). An alternative source is word of mouth. Public sources undoubtedly can contribute far more information than private sources. To the extent that this is true, the quality of the information put into circulation, its objectivity, its timing, and so on, become important factors to consider.

Before reviewing the literature on health planning in the following chapter, one should note that a large share of the health planning literature was produced during the late 1960s and 1970s. If scholarly work reflects to any extent the prevailing values, interpretations, and opinions that exist at the time in society at large, as I have stated in this chapter, then the same must be true of the perspective from which health planning was being considered. Accordingly, historical overviews written during this period tend to portray the medical profession as the primary obstacle to progressive change in the system of health care delivery proposed during the first half of the twentieth century. It is more reasonable to conclude that society was reasonably satisfied with the advances medicine was achieving in the the delivery of health care. Moreover, society was primarily concerned with more pressing economic and social problems (much as it is today) brought about by two major wars and a devastating economic depression.

In sum, the literature which purports to present an objective, data-based evaluation of health planning may, in fact, reflect the larger pattern of social thought prevalent at the time this literature was being produced.

5

Evaluating Health Planning

Over the years evaluations of health planning have become increasingly more sophisticated in their approach and elegant in their form of presentation. The earliest reports were not only less sophisticated and less elegant, they were addressed to a different set of issues. This chapter attempts to capture the perspective from which the problems associated with developing a health planning enterprise were being viewed during the second half of the twentieth century, when health planning entered the era of public sector participation in planning (phase II of the four-phase sequence identified earlier). The review of the literature is organized in chronological order beginning with the years immediately following the enactment of the two initial public sector planning programs—the RMP in 1965 and CHP in 1966. However, this review is not exhaustive, since the amount of material that could be included in such a review is far too extensive. However, the reader is directed to literature reviews which became available at various points in time along the way.

DESCRIBING THE BEGINNINGS OF THE PLANNING EFFORT

One of the earliest references to the health planning legislation that came into existence during this era (RMP and CHP) can be found in the *American Journal of Public Health*. Anticipating the need for guidance in interpreting the new laws, the officials of the American Public Health Association (APHA) published a set of guidelines in the December 1966 issue of the journal. The guidelines advocated including representatives of all relevant agencies in the planning process including health departments, and public and private mental health agencies, welfare departments, and professional schools and voluntary agencies (1966,

2139–2143). The director of the association discussed the guidelines in greater detail in an article in the March, 1967, issue of the journal (Mattison 1967).

Judging from these early discussions in the journal, the members of the APHA generally felt it was incumbent upon them to respond to the new legislation. Because they had been engaged in public health planning all along, they had the most experience to bring to this new stage in health planning for the health needs of the individual. Accordingly, the earliest organized public discussions of the RMP and CHP legislation took place during the APHA meetings in the autumn of 1967. Those who attended the convention seem to have been pleased with the recognition being accorded to the nation's health needs and were eager to begin planning using the newly legislated format (Peterson 1967). A number of the papers presented at these meetings were published in the June, 1968, issue of the journal (vol. 58, 1011–1089). The same issue included an editorial written in response to the confusion about CHP witnessed during the meetings. The editorial interpreted the mandate of CHP as follows. According to the author, the program should encompass: (1) all areas of community health, (2) include all potential resources, (3) but must take into consideration community constraints (for example, norms and attitudes), (4) all of which should be addressed by a formal plan. Having said this the author ended by saying: "the complexity of comprehensive health planning should become less overwhelming" (unsigned editorial, 1968, 1011–1013).

There was little discussion of health planning in the literature during the following year until a number of papers presented during the 1968 annual meetings of the APHA were published in the May, 1969, issue of the journal. Here we find that organizing health planning agencies turned out to be more complicated than anticipated. In fact, the problem confronting persons interested in taking the initial steps in organizing a planning structure were basic indeed. For example, Polk (1969) described how the CHP agency was created in Philadelphia. The first question was: Who should take the initiative and call interested parties together? The second question was: Who should be invited? In Minnesota, similar questions were being asked: Where do we find consumer representatives? (Fifer 1969).

Such questions take on greater significance when the backdrop created by the social context of the time is considered. According to one observer: "Our policy system has remained relatively stable because of the apathetic attitude of the public. We have yet to learn how to operate in a situation where apathy is replaced by such mutual hostility and antagonism toward those in authority" (Feingold 1969, 806). Thus, the focus of early discussions about health planning became fixed on the issue of participation.

A paper presented by Hochbaum (1969), deputy director of the National Center for Health Services Research and Development, during the 1968 APHA meetings outlined the nature of the problems surrounding participation in greater detail. He stated that participation by consumers "holds great promise and many risks." To illustrate, he described a case where a group of disadvantaged consumers

demanded that a category of highly specialized medical specialists be available in their community because they believed that such personnel were available in a wealthy community in the area. When the health professionals argued that the problems these specialists worked on were rare and did not require immediate attention in any case, the community representatives became angry. Hochbaum suggested that the hostility could have been easily avoided if the health professionals had focused on the issue of "equity," pointing out that the services and personnel in question were actually not available in the wealthy community but were located in the medical center hospital. Instead, the health professionals became convinced that the consumers were unreasonable while the consumers saw the episode as evidence that consumer participation was a "coverup" for continued refusal to provide equal care for the disadvantaged.

Hochbaum stated that, while he knew of no instance where consumer participation led to better service than when services were plannned by committed professionals, he believed that consumer participation had to be accepted because this was inevitable. Given this reality, it was important to channel the newly gained sense of power and aggressiveness among consumers, so that constructive contributions would result (1969, 1702). If Hochbaum's message seems harsh from a present-day perspective, perhaps Moore's study documenting the existence of hostility among "indigenous" (poor) consumer representatives can bring the prevailing picture into better focus (1971). She concluded that consumer representatives had little to lose by acting in a hostile manner and, therefore, did act this way whenever they wished to emphasize their point. For a particularly vivid illustration of the prevailing social situation, with which planners had to contend, consider the following commentary on the delivery of services to the poor in Chicago in October, 1969, made by one group interested in planning: "The Black Panther Party is giving a free medical clinic for people who need health care and can't get it from those lousy butcher shop hospitals like Cook County" (Yoder and Reed 1970, 1707).

It is clear that the task of creating a health planning structure from the ground up was a difficult undertaking. The social milieu that prevailed during the late 1960s made the task considerably more complicated. At least part of the aim of some of the participants was to attain greater power and control within the community (Mott 1969; Jonas 1971). Symbolic gains often became as important as more tangible advances in planning, as Hochbaum clearly illustrates (1969). Given the social climate of the time, politicization of health planning was not long in coming (Binstock 1969). Furthermore, politicization was actively advocated by some. Basil Mott observed that planning agencies were being asked to make decisions "that tread heavily upon the toes of important organizations and groups in the health community" without sufficient authority to back up their decisions (1969, 798). He argued that the only avenue planners had available to them was to become good politicians (1969, 799). He criticized the planning models planners were attempting to use at the time, claiming that the "rational decision model," which presents planning as a technical process, was inappro-

priate because a planning technology did not exist, and that the "community action model," which depended on consensus but failed to recognize that there were fundamental differences among the participants involved, was simply naive.

Some, like Avery Colt, placed their trust in sound organizational principles (1969). Colt wanted to see specific goals and criteria identified to permit the measurement and evaluation of goal achievement. One commentator, who apparently assumed that a statistical data base would be required to set goals and later to evaluate progress made in attempting to attain them, waited until the autumn of 1970; then he asked the following question: "Why is it that we [health statisticians] have not been overwhelmed by requests for data from our colleagues in comprehensive health planning?" (Frazier 1970, 1701). With an edge of bitterness, he answered his own question as follows: "Comprehensive health planning in its moribund state has little need for the types of data we usually produce" (1970, 1704). That data problems were not resolved within the next couple of years is apparent in the plea for better data in a paper by Reeves, who concluded his paper by demanding that the APHA support legislation which would assure the availability of necessary data (1972). (It is interesting to note that the federal government did not address seriously the problem of data collection until June, 1978, when it issued national guidelines for planning [Zwick 1978].)

From the perspective of one particularly active committee of the APHA, the main problem stalling effective implementation of CHP was the lack of public awareness about health problems. The Committee on Educational Tasks of the APHA (1970) determined that massive education efforts were required, which should be launched with the cooperation of major educational institutions of all varieties. The education of consumer participants in the planning process continued to be viewed as a pressing problem. A number of reports were published describing consumer training projects, in Berkeley (Parker 1970), in Alabama (Rice 1972), in Chicago (Training for Citizen Participation, n.d.). In discussing the successes and failures of his project, the director of Consumer Training in Alabama ends with the following observation: "In the final analysis, it is obvious that the providers of health services continue to be those most often in attendance in comprehensive health planning meetings. Their interest remains high" (Rice 1972, 979). Observations about consumer versus provider participation were to become more frequent over the years, leading to the generalized belief that the providers dominated consumers, causing health planning to achieve less than it could have were consumers given more control.

There was, at the same time, the continuing struggle to identify the right consumers. Colt pointed out that since everyone consumes health care, everyone is potentially a consumer representative (1970, 1198). He stated that each community would have to determine which consumer representatives fit the needs of the agency in that area. Another problem is revealed by Colt's discussion on consumer selection. When noting that consumers were to constitute the majority, he used the following phrase: "central to the 51 percent requirement" (1970, 1199). In other words, the "majority" required by the law was being literally

interpreted to mean 51%. (The 1974 legislation corrected this misinterpretation by stating explicitly that majority meant 51% to 60 percent.)

Observations on the successes and flaws of health planning do not seem to change very much during the first four to five years that CHP and the RMP were in effect. (For an extensive bibliography of literature on health planning prior to 1971, see Strauss and DeGroot 1971). By 1972 critiques differ only in the specificity of the complaints being mentioned. Roseman, for instance, calls CHP a "scientistic charade" (1972) and advocates replacing the charade of techno-logically based planning with an "overtly political model" (1972, 16). He claimed that greater politicization of staff thinking would overcome a number of specific problems: (1) conflict avoidance, (2) the failure to deal with root causes, (3) the lack of political influence, leadership, and expertise, and (4) grossly inadequate funding (1972, 18). A strikingly similar stance was taken by O'Connor (1974) and Mott (1977).

There were others who were less discouraged by what they observed. Hall, for instance, stated that planning is political and therefore "unavoidably con-troversial" (1972, 75). He described several planning successes. His account was made more interesting by virtue of his willingness to identify his measure of success, which was how closely the consumer participation profile matched the community's profile. While this criterion may not have satisfied everyone, it did serve to focus attention on the fact that measures of success were not being identified by other authors. While this would soon change, we still find papers such as the following, published in 1973. In a brief outline of health planning in their area, a group of planners begin their paper with the following thought: "Seven years have passed and the program though far-reaching in its intent and language . . . has been unable to fulfill its designers' broad vision . . . [sic] it has occurred to the authors that this failure has been the absence of a model for translating the bills' mandate into action programs" (Schwebel et al. 1973). We also find authors advocating an expansion of the health planning mission in the same year (Bruhn 1973). It would appear that after seven or so years of effort, neither those who were observing health planning from the sidelines nor the planners themselves were discouraged even though planning goals were still being debated, and measures of success had not been established. However, this scene was not to last for two reasons; first, evaluation research based on clearly stated measures was in the offing; and, second, the prevailing health planning programs were about to be superseded by a new planning law which would be passed by the end of 1974.

THE ERA OF EMPIRICAL RESEARCH

When Hochbaum addressed the audience during the 1967 APHA meetings, his sense of resignation about accepting consumers into the planning process as a means to calm "the turbulence of restless critics" was balanced by high hope for the solutions forthcoming from social science research. This was the arena in which proper measures would be identified and applied to the benefit of the entire enterprise. He anticipated that the results of "rigorous, factual, and objective research of the social not medical effects" of health planning would have the greatest impact (1969, 1704).

The preceding discussion indicated that a good deal of descriptive material had been collected documenting the start-up difficulties that agencies had experienced. Success stories and disaster stories had been reported. However, empirical studies evaluating the performance of health planning programs had to await the passage of sufficient time so that experience data could accumulate. Reports based on empirical data collected across health planning areas did not become available until the 1970s, when a number of influential reports appeared in rapid succession between 1973 and 1976. Exactly what made these studies influential is worth considering. Clearly, they went beyond describing individual cases by using comparative data. The reports presented tabulated information on selected indicators of performance; and, within the next few years, the data were being treated to quantitative data analysis techniques as well.

What is most impressive about the empirical studies, especially the quantitative research reports, is their ability to organize a massive amount of data, analyze it, and draw clear-cut conclusions based on the objective evidence presented. Another factor distinguishes the empirical studies appearing after 1973 from earlier reports, namely, the indicator used to measure the rate of success in health planning. Not only was it clearly identified, but it reflected the emergent definition of the problem in health care during the early 1970s—the need to control rising health care costs. Thus, as of 1973, the health planning literature split into two branches. The new body of literature focused its attention on evaluating the impact of health planning on health care costs, while the older body of literature continued to address problems surrounding participation in decision making; that is, the earlier body of literature is concerned with the *process* of planning (participation) and the newer branch is concerned with the *outcomes* of planning (cost savings).

Clark Havighurst's analysis of Certificate-of-Need (CON) performance across twenty-three states was one of the first empirical outcome-oriented studies to be published (1973). He found that CON was restricting the supply of services but doing so to the advantage of the bigger, more influential institutions, which he concluded was the same effect that a hospital cartel would have produced. While he questioned the ability of CON to control costs, he concluded that CON review might have had a positive effect on the quality and allocation of services (1973).

William Curran's survey of CON programs currently in operation, published in 1974, provided an important data base documenting the extent of the variation among existing programs. In his 1975 paper, based on the earlier survey, Curran and his co-authors went on to make the observation that once a state begins to impose controls on the health industry, it usually goes on to escalate its regulatory efforts as it finds itself facing resistance (Curran, Steele, and Ober 1975).

The variation in the laws enacted by the state and the stage of development of their planning agencies were found to be directly related to the number of years CON had been in effect by a number of researchers (Certificate of Need 1978). The first CON law was enacted by the state of New York in 1964; by 1970 four other states passed CON legislation. Thus the fact that Curran, Steele, and Ober found twenty-three programs to examine by mid 1974 indicates two facts that must be taken into consideration in reviewing CON performance. First, laws enacted several years apart may be responding to a different social climate; that is, shifting definitions of the problem may be involved. Second, the newer the CON legislation, the less experience the CON agency has had, and, therefore, the less effective it is likely to be. The findings of the Lewin and Associates 1974 study of Section 1122 and CON performance in thirty-six planning areas within twenty states indicated that these two problems did constitute important considerations in evaluating "success." Lewin and Associates found that the states not only varied in performance but, more importantly, varied in what they considered to be their primary objective. Thus the authors reported that the agencies concerned had approved 93% of all projects submitted and 90% of the dollar expenditures proposed (Lewin and Associates 1975, 10). However, the authors also pointed out that "fewer than half of the state and area agencies . . . share the federal commitment to cost containment. Instead, state and local agencies tend to place a much higher priority on improving the quality and distribution of health care resource goals which are sometimes in conflict with cost containment" (Lewin and Associates, 1975, 3).

The assessment carrying the greatest impact was the Salkever and Bice study published in 1976. This was the first quantitative evaluation of CON. The impact of this study can also be attributed to the fact that the findings were so clearly stated and easy to comprehend that they could be widely quoted and discussed. Salkever and Bice concluded that CON did not reduce the dollar amount of investment but did restrict the growth of hospital beds. Investment in expensive technology and its related costs replaced investment in beds. Thus, in the end, there was little impact on the overall per capita cost of hospital care.

A number of other studies published around the same time arrived at similar conclusions. Hellinger (1974), who also used a quantitative methodology, concluded that CON programs did not reduce costs, but that this was due to increased investment in anticipation of CON controls. Katz's (1976) analysis confirmed the fact that CON did not control capital expansion; however, upon closer examination he found that the states experiencing the greatest degree of expansion (of plant assets and beds) were those having the least sophisticated facilities to begin with. (For a thorough critique of the methodological flaws in the studies identified as quantitative research reports plus an extensive annotated bibliography of literature concerned with CON see: Certificate of Need 1978).

At this point, let us examine two related issues in greater detail: first, the approach being used by the empirical data-based studies and, second, the impact these studies have had on the health planning effort. While the research methods employed in these studies are well worth examining, this has been done elsewhere. Instead, let us pursue a line of thought that has not received very much attention. What is most striking in my estimation concerns the timing of the research. Conclusions were reached about the success of cost control efforts before the 1974 legislation, which mandated review of capital expenditures, had been put into operation. Thus, what was being evaluated was the performance of administrative units created prior to 1974—some of which designed to achieve a different purpose (equitable distribution of health care) and others established so recently that they were not fully operative when evaluated. While the studies invariably reported a great deal of variation among the existing CON and Section 1122 programs, they tended, nevertheless, to conclude with a statement on the net effect—a failure to control costs or limit capital expansion. In short, the evaluation research reports published during the mid 1970s did exactly what they purported to do, namely, to evaluate the outcome of health planning to date, using cost control as the criterion of success. Furthermore, they did this using quantitative, that is, objective, data. The flaw is that these studies imposed a measure of success reflecting the outcome that was thought to be desirable during the mid 1970s onto an earlier period of time. The result was an assessment of how well agencies were doing in attaining a goal they did not necessarily espouse.

In 1976 none of the local planning agencies (HSAs) had been "designated," that is, approved, by the federal government. That meant that they did not meet certain government requirements. For example, they did not have a full complement of staff or governing board members, they had been organized inappropriately so they did not represent the community, or had some other shortcomings which prevented them from engaging fully in planning. Lacking full approval meant that they were also not fully funded. Furthermore, federal regulations to guide agencies in making decisions about the appropriate level of services were not available until the later part of 1976. (See Zwick [1978] for an account of the events leading to the publication of guidelines twenty-two months after Congress required that they be issued.) Thus, several types of agencies were combined in evaluation studies including: CHP ''b'' agencies, units created by states to administer CON reviews prior to the 1974 legislation (which set up a uniform set of requirements), and Section 1122 agencies (which also fell under varying administrative units from state to state). After such distinctions were mentioned, evaluation research reports often made inferences about health planning in general rather than any one program or type of agency in particular. Since the existing agencies and the programs under which they were operating were being lumped together, it was not clear whether one program was more effective than another, nor did the fact that some agencies were more successful than others receive much emphasis at the time.

It would not be reasonable to fault researchers who prefer to use large scale data sets for not carrying out in-depth case studies to investigate these differences. However, why other researchers did not attempt to pursue this line of questioning is not clear. Finally, researchers who employed in-depth case analysis methods were largely interested in addressing one dimension of the planning process—problems surrounding participation.

In sum, what one finds in reviewing the literature on health planning is that two bodies of literature exist, one of which is *outcome-oriented* and the other which is *process-oriented*. The primary concerns addressed by one category differ from the primary concerns addressed by the other category; their methods bear little resemblance; with a few exceptions, cross-references to each other's work are infrequent; and, their discussions proceed in mutually exclusive publications. In short, the two bodies of literature generally do not speak to each other.

THE PROCESS-ORIENTED LITERATURE

This section reviews the process-oriented, as opposed to outcome-oriented, literature published as of 1975 which coincides with the first year during which the Health Planning and Development Act legislated in 1974 (PL 93–641) was in operation.

Robert Alford was one of the first to publish a book concerned with the prospects of success that health planning might have for changing the organization of health care (1975). He stated that the difficulties the planning effort had had to date could be attributed to the contradictory aims of the various categories of participants involved. He pointed out that survival of certain institutions often depended on "cooling out" the community because it was the community which tended to be disruptive and therefore posed a threat to survival. Basically, Alford concluded that the likelihood of successful reform was dismal given the institutional barriers created by vested interests.

Another assessment of the health planning enterprise, authored by Herbert Hyman, was also published in 1975. According to Hyman, health planning produced some effects that were not intended. First, a new breed of planners had come into existence, those employed by hospitals were interested in growth, independence, and competition rather than cooperative planning, sharing, and maximizing group needs (1975, 67). Second, government planners were becoming more interested in career security, regular advancement, and pensions rather than promoting more risky, innovative approaches to planning. Hyman also observed that CHP "b" agencies were in the process of transforming themselves into HSAs in response to the 1974 health planning legislation. He presented an assessment of the performance of CHP agencies which he suggested be considered in order to avoid repeating mistakes in organizing the HSAs. His major criticism of the "b" agencies was that they were provider-dominated (1975, 435). He listed the following flaws as well: (1) absence of comprehensive health plans as a framework, (2) incomplete or insufficient criteria for judging proposals, (3) inadequate staff for the quantity and quality of the work load, (4) improperly or underutilized councils or task forces, (5) over-reliance on regulatory process—

neglect of the consultive role, (6) posture of reactive rather than initiative agent, and (7) lack of aggression on commitment to public interest process (1975, 183).

Hyman's treatment of the relationship between CHP agencies and HSAs signaled the beginning of a new era in the literature dealing with the process of planning. What is most striking about this new era is that analyses of the performance of the RMP and CHP continued to be reported long after the two programs had been superseded by the passage of the Health Planning and Development Act of 1974. In fact, evaluations reporting on the achievements of RMP and CHP continued throughout the 1970s. However, these discussions were framed in a context of concern about the newly mandated HSA type of agency. The findings of a number of these studies will be considered.

In examining the upstate New York RMP and CHP, Mott et al. found that, because few accepted standards had evolved, pressing technical issues or professional questions had to be settled, for better or for worse, by vote (1976, 746). Since, according to the authors, this situation was likely to continue even with the new legislation, they concluded that participation continued to be an important issue. Anne and Herman Somers, writing in 1977, concurred: "At the heart of all regulatory systems are the two crucial questions: Who will make the key decisions? How will they be made? These issues are especially critical in the health field, where basic concepts such as measurement of need, quality, and effectiveness are ill defined and disputed, thus leaving wide latitude and discretion to the regulatory bodies" (1977, 241–242).

Addressing the problems faced by any number of programs existing during the 1960s, Lipsky and Lounds also pointed to the lack of specific objectives as well as their instability (1976). The authors claimed that the early attempts to maximize citizen participation tended to conflict with later demands placed on programs, including the need to evaluate programs, to limit spending, to counter internal opposition, and to respond to sponsors' shifting interests. West and Stevens began their assessment by acknowledging that the 1974 legislation corrected a number of problems attributed to the earlier planning programs but, they contended, that the HSAs would encounter many of the same problems faced by the CHP "b" agencies (1976). They predicted that the HSAs would have difficulty "attempting to resist the efforts of organized interests to control the planning agency; obtaining agreement on community-wide goals; defining a balance between sub-area and area-wide interests; preventing organizational issues and project review from dominating the agency's agenda; creating support at the community level; making sure that the council is both representative of and accountable to the public; indicating local power struggles and inter-agency conflicts; and overcoming resistance to change in the health care system" (1976, 194).

While it may appear that there was total consensus with regard to the importance of the participation issue, at least one observer of the scene disagreed. Herbert Klarman (whose training in economics places him in the camp which is generally more interested in the outcome rather than the process of planning) argued that all the concern about participation belied the real problems. He noted: "In the past decade local health planning has been hampered by unstable federal funding. The absence of national policies and guidelines has led to a constant quest for new ideas. In the absence of substantive concerns, requirements for consumer representation have led to a preoccupation with structure and organization" (1976, 1).

Robin MacStravic's study of RMP and CHP performance (1977) reveals an interesting tie between Klarman's assessment of the problem and the concerns of those whom Klarman criticizes. MacStravic found agency size to be the best predictor of performance. (Performance was evaluated according to how closely the agency met the standard of compliance in fulfilling important functions as interpreted by the researchers.) However, there was another dimension to this finding. When the researchers connected size to funding allotment, it became apparent that the larger agencies served bigger populations, meaning that they got more funds from the federal government, which they used to hire more staff; and this was what made it possible to turn out more work.

Although discussion regarding RMP and CHP dropped off after 1976, a few notable examples could be found. We find Drew Altman making the observation in 1978 that PL 93–641 is "a revitalized and refurbished version of this [CHP] earlier health planning program" (1978, 563). This statement precedes a discussion in which Altman outlined the flaws of CHP agencies. In 1979, Luft and Frisvold published a review of the performance of CHP agencies in California. The authors concluded that the CHP agencies could not be effective in controlling costs because the states had not developed a mechanism for reviewing institutional expansion plans (1979, 251).

Louise Russell's influential evaluation of the RMP was released in 1979. She concluded that CHP guidelines were so vague that it was not clear whether the program was interested in promoting or restraining technology. The RMP, by contrast, clearly favored technological expansion. However, it took some time before the "technology of choice" was selected, which turned out to be intensive care technology. Russell's data on this point revealed a high correlation between the money that the particular RMP had available and the number of intensive care beds in the area (1979, 162).

THE EFFECTS OF HEALTH PLANNING EVALUATIONS

After reviewing the early outcome-oriented literature, I suggested that the researchers had made inferences based on their findings which were for various reasons inappropriate. It also appears now that such inferences may have set into motion a snowball effect which had consequences going beyond the initial negative evaluation of health planning. The same thing could be said of the process-oriented evaluations. Some of the process-oriented reports evaluating the performance of the RMP and CHP well after they were no longer in existence made their negative findings more relevant by projecting them onto the newly enacted health planning legislation which created HSAs. This approach increased interest in and the likelihood of publication of what might have otherwise been viewed as outdated research.

Basically, the outcome-oriented researchers found planning to be a failure because it did not succeed in controlling costs; and the process-oriented researchers determined that planning had failed because the participation issue had not been resolved satisfactorily. In combination, these two bodies of literature had a powerful labeling effect. Furthermore, the negative label was applied to the 1974 program while the network of agencies it was mandated to organize was in the earliest stages of development. Whether or not the agencies would have performed any differently if a negative label had not been applied is impossible to determine. What is clear is that the planning effort became stigmatized. How much effect this had on funding further planning efforts is not clear; however, claims that funding was inadequate increased with time (Klarman 1976; Altman 1978; Luft and Frisvold 1979). To what extent the label caused more talented staff members to consider moving to other institutions is also not clear. (Many did move into planning positions in the same hospitals they had been reviewing.) Being labeled a failure may have brought about a series of subtle but corrosive effects that have been observed in a variety of failing enterprises (for example, the railroads). Consider the scenario in which staff members become discouraged; the providers and consumers, who serve in a voluntary capacity, become less willing to sacrifice their time and energy; the institutions to be regulated become less willing to assume a conciliatory stance, choosing instead to evade or bypass the regulatory agency's procedures whenever possible.

This dismal scenario did not develop overnight. However, it did develop in some instances (in the HSA I studied, for example), and it is likely that the stigma of failure played a part in promoting such a scenario. Furthermore, no one rebutted the label, at least not in print. Even those who favored planning found much to criticize. Bruce Vladek's (1981) relatively recent comments provide a good illustration. In an earlier statement he began his comments by saying: "In government, anatomy is destiny" (1977, 83). He continued: "The effective result is change of only the most incremental, meliorist sort." The structure outlined by PL 93–641, he argued, simply "provides an institutional forum for legitimizing existing patterns of power distribution" (1977, 27). Also, there is the suggestion that Vladek finds some communality with Klarman, who stated that all the attention being focused on participation masked the real problem (1977). According to Vladek, the real problem was the lack of "detailed specification of the kinds of activities HSAs are to conduct. Attention therefore necessarily turns to specifying the individuals who are to be involved in the process" (1977, 28).

Basil Mott (1977) seems to be in complete agreement with Vladek. He stated that health planning agencies faced a near-impossible task for three reasons: (1) the anatomy of health planning, (2) the limited means available to health planning agencies to make meaningful changes in the behavior of health care providers, and (3) the institutional character of the health field (1977, 244). He also lamented the lack of a rational basis for decision making (1977, 249) as did Vladek (1977, 28). Klarman also made the point that such measures were especially important under the circumstances, since we have no experience to date in carrying out a "policy of contraction" (1978, 109).

Reporting the results of a project examining the relationship between planning and regulation, Bauer stated:

Up to now, planners' efforts towards better allocation and organization of health services in their area have met with no greater success than regulators' efforts to control the rising costs of institutional services. However, were the pot itself to be constrained . . . the planners' approach to managing changes in the system could well prove to be more successful over the long run than the regulators' hard fought case-by-case decisions. (1978, 6)

Apparently the partnership between planning and regulation worked well in some areas, Rhode Island, for example (Bauer 1978, 6) and at cross-purposes in other areas, as in Maryland (Altman 1978, 572). According to other observers the relationship between planning and regulation will never work. Wildavsky took this position:

Planning, as I have said, is being able to control the future through present acts. . . . Control of the future demands knowledge (understanding what one does) and power (compelling others to accomplish one's will). [Wildavsky says planners have neither knowledge nor power.] But to have planning does not require a plan. Any process of decision that effects behavior, whether it is a market or administrative mechanism, may be thought of as a plan. . . . Planning need not be a single solution; it can be, and often is, a convoluted way of restating the problem: can we increase the quantity and quality of medical services while decreasing costs? The answer is, we can't. (1979, 302)

The conclusion reached by Bauer (1978), namely, that the "pot" must be constrained, was being reached by others as well. By the close of 1984, eleven states plus a larger number of individual Blue Cross plans had introduced "rate setting" or "prospective reimbursement" programs which set limits on hospital revenue for the year (McIlrath 1984, 1). Early evaluations gave this approach a mixed review (Biles, Schramm, and Atkinson 1980); however, an increasing number of reports indicated that it could be a highly successful mechanism of control once fully operative (Bauer 1977; for review see Lefkowitz 1983). Additional studies have recently been commissioned in response to concerns that prospective payment may be threatening care to the elderly (McIlrath 1985).

During the same period some were arguing on behalf of stricter regulation in the form of prospective payment to hospitals, the ranks of those advocating that the planning enterprise be dismantled and replaced by a market solution were also beginning to expand. (These critiques laid the foundation for programs launched during the current health planning phase.) Some of the more commonly cited proponents of this argument include Havighurst (1978), Enthoven (1981),

Feldstein (1981), McClure (1981), and the Congressional Budget Office (1982). (For extended discussion and debate on competition versus regulation also see Greenberg [1978]; Zubkoff, Raskin, and Hanft [1978]; and Ginzberg [1982].)

By the late 1970s the general consensus was that health planning had not produced the impact expected; as a result, the 1974 planning act was amended in 1979 in an effort to correct some of the problems critics had pointed out. One of the major points of clarification was directed at specifying the criteria for selecting consumer representatives. The amendment also advocated "batching" CON reviews in order to compare proposals concerned with similar plans. Review of computerized axial tomography (CAT) scanners was removed from the list of reviewable services. The threshold was raised from $150,000 to $600,000 for considering projects reviewable. Six additional planning priorities were specified. However, the effect of this amendment was short-lived; whether the amendment would have had a greater effect in the long run is difficult to determine since the social climate was on the verge of another major shift. Health planning was about to be swept into the groundswell of sentiment favoring the reduction of federal control and regulatory intervention. With Reagan's election to the presidency in 1980 came cuts in funding of governmental regulatory activities in the health sector as he had promised during his campaign for office. While the Health Planning and Development Act (PL 93–641) is still in effect at the time this is being written, funding cuts have been so drastic that the planning agencies can do very little of what they were originally expected to accomplish.

EVALUATION OF HEALTH PLANNING IN THE 1980s

Even though health planning did not look as if it would survive much past 1980, evaluations of the performance of the 1974 planning act continued to appear in the 1980s (Fotion 1985). A major report was issued under the auspices of the Institute of Medicine in 1981. In the preface of the first of the two-volume report, Rashi Fein, who chaired the review committee, stated:

No program can succeed if it is constantly subjected to changing guidelines, altered priorities, and mixed signals. Nor is morale enhanced if the program and the required appropriations are constantly in jeopardy. It is possible to ensure failure by underfunding programs, harassing administrators, showing little appreciation for thousands of citizens involved, and setting unattainable goals. (1981, viii)

Fein also made clear the sense of the committee regarding the value of planning in his opening statement: "Does the contribution that health planning makes and can make . . . justify the effort? This committee is convinced that the answer to that question is yes" (1981, vii). In addition to summarizing the views of the committee members and findings presented in the commissioned papers, published as volume two, the first volume also presented an historical overview of the development of planning agencies. Thus, we find that only nine out of the

205 agencies planned were fully "designated" (federally approved) by 1978, and that 171 were fully designated by February of 1979 (1981, 23). We are referred to the committee's first-year report on the standards and guidelines governing planning, where the committee reported the difficulties incurred by agencies expected to operate without planning guidelines that were issued almost two years after the PL 93–641 was enacted (Institute of Medicine 1980). The central thrust of the report, however, is addressed to the health planning process. The problems surrounding participation served as the main topic of discussion in eight of the ten commissioned papers published in volume two. The two papers which do not address participation are by Downs, who discusses measurement problems (1981, 89–113), and by Cohodes, who reviewed the success of capital expenditure controls (1981, 54–88).

The remaining eight papers gave health planning a less than glowing review. In the two papers Checkoway contributed, he argued for the professionalization of consumers via resource mobilization, that is, developing career opportunities, which he said worked well in the agencies he examined (1981, 157–183; 184–203). Morone, in the first of two papers, advocated correcting the consumer participation problem by ensuring that the consumers would be accountable to the specific constituency they were to represent (1981, 225–256). In the second paper, Morone presented a tongue-in-cheek characterization of HSA participants (1981, 257–289). Raab identified another set of actors—those involved in the governmental in-fighting that was responsible for certain aspects of the final design of PL 93–641 (1981, 114–142). After giving planning a lukewarm evaluation, Brown stated that "debating, deliberating, and consensus-building" is fruitful even if it does not produce success (1981, 1–53). In contrast, Sapolsky claimed that success would never be attained unless a limit was placed on capital expenditures, and allocation of capital was placed in the hands of payers and consumers (1981, 143–156). Ellenburg went even further by advocating real "consumer control," not simply consumer participation (1981, 204–224).

In general, the process-oriented literature published in the 1980s found the participation issue still unresolved. The concept of "imbalanced political markets" emerged as a prominent theme (Marmor and Morone 1980; Checkoway 1981; Checkoway, O'Rourke, and Macrina 1981; Morone 1981). In effect, the general conclusion reached by the process-oriented researchers has been that health planning as a whole has not succeeded. Whether this assessment is due entirely to the determination that the participation issue was not satisfactorily resolved is not clear, for a number of reasons. To begin with, no agreed-upon indicator of successful as opposed to unsuccessful participation in the health planning decision-making process has emerged. Instead, what tends to stand in for evidence is the statement that providers dominated consumers. However, careful reading of this body of literature does not provide much direct evidence of provider domination (one exception to this generalization can be found in Altman, Greene, and Sapolsky 1981, 26–31.) As far as I can see, this assessment has often been made by researchers who based their judgments about process on the evidence which refers to the outcome. In other words, if consumers agreed with providers, it must be because they were being dominated. However, if participation for the sake of participation in the decision-making process was thought to be valuable in and of itself, how can consumer participation be regarded as a failure? After all, consumers were in the majority and they did participate—unless they did not accomplish what they were expected to accomplish for which someone—the providers—had to be blamed. This assessment apparently has had such broad appeal that there has been little sense of need to examine it more closely.

The outcome-oriented researchers have identified a longer list of reasons for the lack of success. Thus, the composite picture presented by both categories of researchers of the health planning record through 1980 was clearly a negative one. Therefore, when it came, the reversal in the conclusions reached by the outcome-oriented evaluators was totally unexpected. To illustrate, Cain states that an examination of U.S Census Bureau figures indicates that "annual expenditures for facilities construction, in constant dollar terms, fell by 26% from 1976 to 1979" (1981, 165). Howell's research indicates that hospitals in Massachusetts were in a phase of extensive expansion between 1967 and 1976, but during that time CON review reduced the scale and cost of projects being proposed by "as much as two-thirds" (1981). In fact, a comprehensive review of the most recent evaluation reports indicates that a small but convincing body of evidence has accumulated showing that the CON review process did have a positive effect on slowing the rate of capital expenditure (Stiles, 1983).

The revised assessment of health planning effects that has come from the outcome-oriented researchers has produced a far more complicated picture than the one that existed prior to the 1980s. Added to the impact produced by this reversal is the fact that the issues addressed separately by the two branches of the health planning literature seem to be converging. For example, one observation that has become widely accepted is that the states, as well as the individual HSAs, varied greatly in how they performed, particularly with regard to control over capital expenditures. This has largely been attributed to the extensive variation in the degree to which planning agencies chose to commit themselves to federal planning goals (Lewin 1975; Altman, Greene, and Sapolsky 1981; Little 1982; Stiles 1983). It is now clear that the states confronting the need to contain health care costs years ago not only had the advantage of a firm commitment to the federal cost containment goal, but had accumulated a considerable amount of experience in utilizing the mechanisms created to attain that goal as well.

It is now also more apparent that success was less than complete even in these cases because the avenues around such controls were being developed with a similarly high level of speed and commitment. We find, for example, that though the federal government had abolished the Hill–Burton program, institutions were able to obtain subsidized loans for capital expenditure purposes from the Federal Housing Administration, the Small Business Administration, the Economic Development Administration, and the Farmer's Home Administration (Altman,

Greene, and Sapolsky 1981, 6). This is also the period of time during which a variety of other new and creative financing methods evolved (Cohodes and Kinkead 1984). In addition, Lefkowitz notes that eighty-five direct loans plus 281 loan guarantees were still outstanding in the Hill–Burton portfolio as of 1981 (1983, 167).

Most observers are in agreement with regard to the reasons behind the variation in level of commitment to federal planning goals across planning areas. These include differences in political characteristics, public support, local incentive structures, coordination with other programs, and program maturity (Stiles 1981). I expect that many, if not all, observers would also agree with Bonnie Lefkowitz's (1983) recent assessments. She determined that a major factor is the direction from which the planning impetus comes: that the states which opted for a "top-down approach" toward planning based on regulation and the imposition of constraints fared better than states which employed a "bottom-up approach" based on voluntarism and pluralism.

Yet pluralism could not always be avoided, particularly in situations when residents of the community were opposed to any restrictions in service. Pluralism was also more likely to have played a part when the benefits of specific procedures were not yet fully explored but which the public was convinced were especially promising.

The CAT scanner issue is perhaps the perfect example of the interaction between the analytical and political aspects of health planning. Planners are faced with a problem, the rapid proliferation of technology that is both expensive to purchase and to operate. Demand is guaranteed; the manufacturers market aggressively and physicians, patients, and hospitals act as eager, affluent consumers. Although health planners need to act quickly, cost/benefit data and information are insufficient and inconclusive. Indeed, given the value questions involved in assessing benefits, the data are likely to remain inconclusive. Planners adapt by adjusting the regulatory response incrementally, attempting to slow the introduction of new scanners while soliciting further information. This policy of gradualism is formalized in numerical standards and guidelines. (Altman, Greene, and Sapolsky 1981, 127)

In the final analysis, the consensus seems to be that health planning turned out to have been effective where people were committed to a health planning approach for containing health care costs. Where people were not committed to the goal of cost containment in general and restraint of capital expenditures in particular, health planning was not effective. This interpretation leaves little reason for assuming that any alternative approach would have proved more effective.

CONCLUSION

The evaluations of planning programs became more sophisticated in their approach and elegant in their presentation over time, and outcome-oriented literature, which largely focused on the impact of CON review on cost containment, did indeed become highly sophisticated. However, even more important is that the conclusions presented in this branch of the literature have gone through a complete reversal between the mid 1970s and the early 1980s. While the earlier evaluations determined that existing capital expenditure controls were ineffective, more recent evaluations report that planning agencies succeeded in containing the rising costs of health care to a greater extent than earlier studies had indicated. The other major branch of the literature, which addresses the process of planning, found the planning endeavor to be flawed from its beginnings and has not reversed that assessment between the late 1960s and early 1980s.

There are a number of reasons to explain the reversal on the assessment regarding planning outcomes: (1) early studies based this assessment on the performance of agencies which were not fully established, (2) agencies operating under the auspices of different programs were lumped together so that conclusions were generalized to the entire planning enterprise rather than any one program, (3) agency performance measures were not well developed, and (4) major differentiating characteristics across agencies were not considered, such as the quality or age of existing capital stock (buildings and beds).

In contrast to the outcome-oriented literature, the process-oriented literature did not alter its early assessment of the problems inherent in the health planning process based on later evidence. The earliest reports began by describing the difficulties agencies had in trying to establish themselves. This was followed by discussions identifying specific problems and documentation of the steps taken by individual agencies in overcoming such problems. The dominant theme emerging in these early discussions concerned the problems surrounding participation in the decision-making process. This topic has continued to provide the central focus of discussion in the process-oriented branch of the planning literature throughout the 1970s and into the 1980s.

If the flaws attributed to the outcome-oriented literature can be listed in an orderly manner, it is because this portion of the literature has been extensively reviewed and criticized (Certificate of Need . . . 1978; Stiles 1983). The process-oriented literature has not benefited by such treatment. My criticism of the latter body of literature primarily has been directed at the portion published during the mid to late 1970s. While the reports published during this period were based on evidence gathered on RMP and CHP, which were no longer operative, these reports were framed in larger discussions concerned with the newly emerging HSAs created by the 1974 legislation. Thus, this body of literature can be faulted for projecting the flaws found in the performance of one set of agencies onto another generation of agencies operating under the auspices of an entirely different program even before those agencies were fully established.

The effect of negative evaluations of planning outcomes as well as the planning process was to cast the entire planning endeavor in an unfavorable light. This resulted in a self-fulfilling prophecy. Thus, the conclusions of the most recent outcome-oriented evaluations are all the more remarkable, since they report that health planning must be credited for controlling a considerably greater share of health care costs than earlier research had indicated. More to the point, these cost savings were achieved under conditions which were less than ideal.

In the final analysis, I would like to make more explicit the implications drawn from these conclusions. At this point I am less interested in arguing on behalf of planning as the best mechanism of control over the health care system and more interested in considering the impact that program evaluation may have on a program's future prospects. Scientific, objective, and well-intended evaluations can still have damaging effects if their findings are not judiciously interpreted and their recommendations cautiously tested before being fully embraced.

The fact that evaluation research is itself developing into a minor industry also must not be overlooked. Some observers are arguing that this enterprise is not likely to survive given that federal funding of health services research has been severely cut (Friedman 1984). However, this may have the undesirable effect of intensifying competition for those funds, thereby exacerbating an already highly competitive situation. It has been true for some time that as the vested interests of the evaluation research organizations and individual evaluators have become more entrenched, survival has become a more salient issue, and, in turn, gaining greater recognition has risen in importance as the means to that end. The temptation to be the first to publish an evaluation report on the performance of a new program is now being spurred on by more practical concerns than prestige. If one does not manage to be the first, there are some alternatives. A high level of recognition can be attained (assuming, of course, that interest in the program remains high) if one presents evidence reversing the findings of earlier reports. As we have seen, evaluation research, which is completed after the program is already in decline, can be made relevant if it can be connected to a new program in the offing.

In embarking on an evaluation research project one simply takes one's chances because it is not always easy to predict what will happen to the program while the research is being carried out. Consider the time involved in writing the proposal for funding, waiting for the funding agency to review it, collecting the data, analyzing the data, writing up the findings, and getting the report into print. Clearly, the career of a researcher can be significantly affected by the timing and selection of the program to be evaluated. This is true of individuals in academia as well as those associated with independent research and/or consulting firms. After investing many months or years of effort, one does not abandon the work easily without trying to salvage as much of it as possible, even if the program involved is no longer as important as it was when the research was initiated.

Beyond the self-interest of researchers is the pressure applied by interest groups on government representatives who, in turn, expect program administrators to provide evidence that the program has performed well or the opposition to show that it has not. The rise and fall of programs depends to a large extent on the public's reaction and the media's presentation of such reports.

The concatenation of health planning measures discussed here was, to some extent, the result of a similar set of pressures. Consider the pattern they present. The health planning programs of the 1960s were enacted together with a large number of other programs intended to address one set of public demands (increased access); during the 1970s, the same programs found themselves being faulted for not addressing a revised set of demands (cost containment). The urgency of the latter problem put a premium on the length of time allotted to the prevailing program before the cries for abandoning it for lack of results were heard. Similarly, the Health Planning and Development Act (PL 93–641) has been superseded by an even newer approach in the form of the Diagnostic Related Groups Program (DRG) enacted in 1982 as an amendment to Medicare legislation (the Tax Equity and Financial Responsiblity Act, PL 97–248). (For a review of the origins of this legislation see Dunham and Morone 1983.) This program was enacted largely on the basis of positive evaluation reports based on the experience of one state, New Jersey. However, the positive reports were themselves being challenged before this new program was fully operative—indeed, even before completion of the first year of this program's three-year phase-in period (Iglehart 1982; Wennberg, McPherson, and Caper 1984). In fact, some observers have called for the program to be abandoned. Walter McClure has been quoted as saying: "Scrap DRGs and replace it with this [rate-setting]" (McIlrath 1984, 41).

It should not be surprising to see the pattern witnessed during the life of earlier planning programs repeated during the next few years. Initially, the DRG program was highly lauded as an exciting and innovative mechanism of control over rising costs. Once the program was enacted, reports began to appear indicating that it was not as successful as it originally appeared to be. Using past experience as a guide, this should lead to a casting about for an alternative mechanism of control well before this program is fully established. Finally, years later, once there are longitudinal experience data, researchers may find that this program too worked better, in specific cases, than initial reports suggested. In order to forestall this sequence of events, a commission (the Prospective Payment Assessment Commission) has been established to study and recommend necessary adjustments in the DRG program. It is also worth noting that Stuart Altman, who has been appointed as chairman of this commission, has observed: "It is inconceivable that at the first crack you will come up with a perfect system. I think the test of this system over the next five to ten years will be willingness of the federal government to make appropriate changes to make it work better" (1984, 104). It is impossible not to wonder whether Altman will have that much time before new approaches are initiated.

The literature reviewed in this chapter indicates that much has been learned over the past three decades about the health care delivery system, the components involved, their pattern of development, and, most importantly for purposes of this discussion, something about why attempts to control the system have proved effective in some instances and not in others. However, little found in this body of literature reflects a sociological perspective. The literature has a great deal to say about participation in the process of planning and about the dollar value of planning outcomes. What is lacking is attention to the effects that the structural dimension may have had on planning efforts. The interactions I observed, as well as the responses I received to the questions I posed in interviewing HSA participants in carrying out this study, reveal a number of stress points in agency structure. Thus, in the following three chapters I consider my findings in light of the conclusions found in the existing literature; analyze my observations from a sociological perspective; and show how the application of sociological insight could have predicted some of the difficulties encountered by those involved in the planning endeavor.

Part II
The Urban HSA

6

The Participants' Evaluation of Success

Permission to conduct this case study was granted to me by the Urban HSA based on my intention to answer the following question: "What have we learned from the health planning experience?" I expected to answer this question by participating in the work being done by the governing board and by the CON Committee (one of the four task force committees in existence at the time) as well as by interviewing the participants. The staff members who worked with the members of both the committee and the board included me in the process of reviewing proposals, writing staff reports, making site visits, and presenting staff evaluations during committee and governing board meetings. The data collection process lasted for twenty months, beginning in January, 1982.

The data are based on interviews with thirty-three persons (thirty of whom were voting members plus three ex-officio representatives of interested organizations in the area, such as the Veterans Administration Hospital) currently serving on the CON Committee and the governing board. Many individuals served on both the committee and the board. Each of these persons was asked to answer four questions: (1) How did you happen to become involved with the Urban HSA? (2) Do you feel you represent a particular constituency? (3) If you had to evaluate the HSA's performance on a scale of one through five (five being high), how would you rate it? (4) Knowing what we know now, what could the HSA have done differently? Each question was followed by additional probing questions to encourage the individual to expand on his or her answers. By the time we got to the fourth question, people were generally surprised to find that they had so much to say. In this chapter I will review the answers to questions 3 and 4. (Chapter 7 discusses questions 1 and 2. Observational data recorded during meetings are discussed in chapter 8.)

This chapter examines the characteristics distinguishing the consumer representatives from the provider representatives. More specifically, the discussion addresses the extent to which participants differ in their understandings of the Urban HSA's purpose, estimates of its success, and ideas regarding what it could do to attain a greater level of success. The primary aim here is to explore assumptions regarding the differences between the two categories of participants. As the discussion proceeds, it should become increasingly more obvious that the attitudes held by the Urban HSA participants differ from the picture painted of both consumers and providers by the existing literature. The data indicate that basic differences do exist between the two regarding the impact that health planning could be expected to have on the health care delivery system. However, these data also reveal the existence of a far greater degree of diversity in the attitudes held by individuals within each of the two categories regarding actual achievements of the planning effort, the health care system in general, and the decision makers who represent health care institutions.

Previous research, especially that portion identified as the process-oriented branch of the literature, is grounded in the belief that providers can invariably be expected to favor attempts to expand the health care delivery system and that consumers can just as invariably be expected to oppose it. The discussion here challenges these expectations by reporting participants' statements regarding the attitudes they hold, the strengths and weaknesses they feel they bring to this effort, as well as some clues as to their motivation for participating in the work of the Urban HSA.

I do not wish to suggest that my observations can be generalized to apply to other HSAs. The individuals involved in other HSAs—the governing board members, executive directors, committee members, and staff—all contribute to each agency's particular character and performance. Each HSA is located in an area having a different population from other areas, a different set of institutions, a different record of health-seeking behaviors, and so on. Therefore, it is not intended that the patterns of interaction, structures, and evaluations identified here are treated as if they were typical. Instead, my hope is that this account is sufficiently provocative to challenge a number of assumptions that have become firmly embedded in the belief system surrounding the general health planning record of performance.

THE DIFFERENCES IN VIEWS AMONG PARTICIPANTS

When asked how successful they thought the HSA had been on a scale of one (low) through five (high), the consumers (n = 17) gave it a mean score of 3.4 with a modal rating of 4. The providers (n = 13) rated it at 2.4 with a modal score of 2. The reason behind such a wide margin of difference became more apparent in the answers that the respondents gave to the next question they were asked to answer. I asked: "Knowing what we know now, what could the HSA have done differently?" The responses came in the form of complaints about problem areas as well as expressions of pride about accomplishments. Providers listed the following points of frustration (in order of frequency): (1) The law itself was not well designed, which created problems in application; (2) the role of the state was duplicative of the work performed by the local HSA, sometimes reversing the HSA's decisions with no explanation; and (3) one of the major health care problems, rising costs, was outside of the HSA's control. Two tasks that some providers thought might be accomplished better were collecting more and better data and developing a more workable health plan. Other functions that the HSA should fulfill but had not done very well according to one or two people included providing better training for participants, especially the consumers; disseminating the data collected by the HSA to providers in the area; developing better public education programs; and identifying clear measures of success. A few providers added that they had little hope of any success as long as some of the major institutions in the area were not prepared to cooperate with the HSA and with each other.

The two activities mentioned most frequently by consumers as activities the HSA should improve upon were increased public education and providing better education for the participants, especially the consumers. Tied for third place were the sense of frustration caused by the state agency's veto power over the HSA's decisions and the sense of defeat caused by the recently approved cuts in federal funding. Two mentions went to the lack of a clarity in the law and the failure to develop a better health plan for the city. Finally, individuals expressed dissatisfaction with inadequacies in the following areas: data collection, evaluation measures of success, and clarification of what the HSA was expected to accomplish. Two consumers said they were disappointed because the agency had not attended to issues they felt should have been priorities— preventive care and finding cures for the major diseases.

At the same time, the consumers found more to be satisfied about than the providers. The greatest source of satisfaction came from the sense that they personally had learned a great deal. The HSA's efforts to open up the process of health care planning to the public was mentioned by virtually every consumer as a laudable achievement. A couple of people said that they were pleased with the agency's efforts to educate the public. Several people cited with pride certain documents produced by the HSA. Finally, two people indicated a certain amount of satisfaction based on their affiliation with the HSA because, they said, if it had not been for the HSA "things would have been worse."

The providers found fewer reasons to be satisfied. Three persons stated that the HSA had done a good job in educating the public. Two saw success in the fact that the consciousness of hospital administrators had been raised. One mention each went to the agency's data collection efforts, its ability to encourage open participation in health planning and finally the feeling that "things would have been worse" if not for the HSA.

Clearly, there is some consensus among the participants regarding the agency's successes and failures. To the extent that the respondents sought to attribute blame for the agency's inability to achieve an even higher level of success, the state agency and the federal government provided ready targets. Also, neither the consumers nor the providers were sparing of their fellow participants or the staff in passing around the responsibility for the lack of greater success.

The providers' view of the role played by consumers can be summed up as a combination of understanding at the intellectual level and a considerable amount of impatience at the practical level. Statements made by a number of providers illustrate this.

Sometimes the consumers go off in weird directions. But that's okay; they have to ask the questions they want answered.

It has been terribly frustrating, at least in the early days. We would spend half of every meeting explaining general background information. You have to have an informed vote. Then the committee memberships would change and periodically it was necessary to do it again. They didn't know what a single room was; why you would want one—not that it's luxurious or special, but some kinds of medical problems require it. You have to educate people in the language, the concepts, what it takes to do the job. Like why it takes us 4.6 nurses for one neo-natal intensive care unit patient. Yes, it takes that many nurses; you have to explain why to people. Informed decision making requires that knowledge. From the perspective of the consumers, they thought that this knowledge came down from their promethean ancestors. That was really a bummer!

Their actions are often arbitrary, unreasoning. I know that they are voting and they don't know what they're voting on. It is not adequate to turn this activity over to the mob. This isn't the French Revolution.

The notion that consumers were asking bothersome questions was by and large the sense that came through the statements of most providers. There were, however, a few providers who took the opposite stance, as the statement of one provider, a physician, illustrates:

I have not seen an example of a consumer majority imposing an unwise decision on providers. I have seen them adding to this, a dimension of decision making in a healthy way.

It is not surprising that the providers who answered very basic questions about highly sophisticated pieces of equipment and services based on complex diagnostic and treatment techniques ended up concluding that the consumers, whom they were teaching, were far from being adequately informed to make decisions that carried very serious consequences. The response of consumers to their lack of knowledge undoubtedly played a part in shaping provider attitudes toward this format for making decisions about health care delivery arrangements. To illustrate, one consumer representative's attitude regarding the amount of background information required to make a decision was indicated in the following tale which he told about himself: "I didn't know about some of these things. All during one meeting, they kept talking about a CAP [sic] scanner. Finally, I went up to [the president of the executive board] and said, 'What's a CAP scanner?' She told me. So then it was okay.'' This person felt that he was then adequately prepared to make the kind of judgment he was being asked to make. He also admitted that he agreed to serve on this committee without being interested in the agency's purpose or having much knowledge about matters of health. He was invited to accept the position because he was a well known community leader from an underserved community. This consumer's sense of confidence provided a sharp contrast to the tentativeness with which such decisions were treated by other HSA members.

One unusually conscientious consumer representative who was an experienced administrator but who had decided to take some time off before taking on a new challenge, stated the following concerns: "There is so little time to consider these complicated proposals. I have often had questions but didn't ask them. Then I've gone home and said to myself, 'now why didn't you do that?' ''

A number of consumer representatives mentioned that an orientation session would help to deal with the knowledge gap problem. Consumers who had been around for a longer period of time recalled how valuable their initial orientation had been and regretted that funds were no longer available for such a program.

There were also a number of providers who felt less than fully qualified to deal with some of the issues they were asked to confront. One provider stated: "A lot of the committee members aren't interested in all of these things. For example, I don't feel competent to vote on CAT scanners." She observed that people dealt with their strengths and weaknesses in a variety of ways. She added this illustration based on her experience working with another Urban HSA committee earlier to make her point: "Even though the staff repeatedly instructed us not to be concerned about the budget but to consider the appropriateness and need for the services, several committee members picked away at the budget. That's because they felt more comfortable talking about these things."

THE STRENGTHS AND WEAKNESSES OF PARTICIPANTS

There is no question that the providers were usually in the position of supplying technical information and the consumers were in the position of having to ask for explanations. Such a division of labor does seem to lend support to the widespread belief that the providers dominate the health planning process. However, this assumes that technical information, even intentionally biased explanations intended to persuade consumers to agree with the providers, will have a more powerful impact than the values that the consumers, as individuals, bring to bear on the process. Consider the following statements by consumers, starting with one consumer's views about the major medical center adjacent to his community:

They've got a Who's Who sitting up in their offices. Some of these hospitals have golf courses, spas, saunas, and the poor patients are paying for it. . . . They're no different than A.T. & T. The only difference is that they're non-profit, which means they can accept contributions. If anybody thinks' hospitals are losing money, that's a myth. They've got administrators up there over [that is, in charge of] water coolers. You mean they're losing money? They get competent administrators so they can put lies on paper accurately.

Another consumer, whose view of providers was considerably less hostile, enjoyed a hearty chuckle recalling the position that he and the ad hoc voting block to which he was recruited took during one meeting:

I remember at the first meeting we burned two hospitals. [The executive director of the agency] was jumping up and down because under the rules, they could get the new beds they wanted. But, we thought, if they grab it all, it'll leave nothing for everybody else.

To even the balance, at least in these examples, there were also consumers who held a very sympathetic view of providers and health institutions:

The hospitals need everything they're asking for. Everywhere they're building. It's hard. After you see these projects, they're at capacity; I don't see any waste. They don't have any waste.

The question is to what extent is technical information or persuasion by providers likely to affect the predispositions of these individuals? I will not speculate about the answer. However, I do want to note that the values people bring to such a process may play a larger role than has been recognized to date. Furthermore, the participants bring to this process a very wide range of strengths and weaknesses both in terms of their knowledge and their personal characteristics. Some are knowledgeable about health care delivery from a medical standpoint, others from an administrative and financial standpoint; there are some who are experienced in the delivery of health care in the community rather than in hospitals; still others are better acquainted with the needs of specific categories of consumers, for example, the aged or the disabled. In other words, no one could possibly be an expert in all areas. There is no question that some participants were more knowledgeable than others; however, this posed less of a problem than the fact that some participants were also unfamiliar with formal meeting procedures. The rules governing meeting behavior had to be explained repeatedly for the benefit of one or two consumers, which not only caused a certain amount of discomfort, but cast doubt on the ability of these individuals to make informed decisions regarding the content of the discussion.

Beyond differences in technical knowledge and meeting procedures, there were personality differences affecting how aggressive various individuals were, how responsible they were in preparing for meetings, whether they had a personal set of objectives they were trying to meet via the HSA, and so forth. During the time I worked with the HSA, there were any number of occasions during which the participants had the opportunity to display common human foibles. To illustrate, when television cameras were brought in to record a particularly newsworthy meeting, a number of those present responded as if they were auditioning for a part in a continuing series. A few people volunteered to be interviewed after the meeting. One was, in fact, selected. Another person, who was obviously enjoying the media attention, positioned herself so she would be in full view of the camera, seemingly oblivious to the fact that she was then sitting in the center of the room with her back to the chairman.

There were numerous occasions for other less than flattering stereotypes of group decision making to be played out. For example, when one institution's proposal for building an extensive parking facility came up for review, many more people than usual had something to add to the discussion. It was difficult to observe this set of proceedings and not be reminded of one of Parkinson's laws (1957). Parkinson illustrates this particular law by describing the proceedings of a university committee meeting called to review two campus construction projects, one a $300 bicycle shed and the other a multimillion-dollar nuclear physics building. The plans for the physics building passed unanimously, while the bicycle shed inspired lengthy debate. The difference, according to Parkinson, was that everyone had some experience with projects of the bicycle-shed variety; in contrast to their experience with nuclear physics buildings. Not being sure what questions to ask and not wishing to embarrass themselves, they passed it without comment. The parallel here is obvious.

What motivates HSA participants to behave as they do is the topic of Jim Morone's (1981) tongue-in-check analysis. He presents the following typology. Among providers Morone finds four types:

1. Neanderthal—government has no place in medicine.
2. Self-seekers—providers (often administrators) who use planning to their own (institution's) ends.
3. Tory—cautious reform to avert revolutionary change.
4. Renegade—dedicated to health planning or cost containment or other innovations that might alter the organization, financing, or practice of medicine.

Among the consumers Morone identifies six types:

1. Eminents and warm bodies—many eminents are too busy; others are not sufficiently interested. They rarely understand what membership entails.
2. Volunteers—advocates without a cause, seeking to do some communal good.
3. Advocates—take a systematic "public interest" view with a clear vision of the changes they wish to introduce.
4. Interest group champions—interested in the advantages for their constituency.
5. Occupational representatives—speak for organizations that employ them, usually unions, insurers, and large companies.
6. Statesmen and politicians—have few referents outside, but focus on the agency, its process, its politics. (1981, 262–270)

It is easy to find amusement in the performance of people in groups of all sorts. HSA participants are not unique on this dimension. In fact, when one considers the complexity of the assignment that HSA participants were asked to accept as volunteers, it is easier to understand why they might be tempted to seek approval and recognition for their efforts within the group and on occasion from outsiders via the media. (A few of the participants from both the consumer and provider categories agreed to talk to me for similiar reasons. This became clear when I stated that they could speak freely because I would not attribute anything that was said to individuals. They responded by urging me to use their names in what I expected to write.)

STAFF ASSISTANCE

During the HSA's first few years, committee members received a copy of the proposal, together with its supporting materials, plus a staff evaluation which could run into hundreds of pages. The xeroxing and mailing costs were enormous, and the committee members complained about the volume of material they were expected to digest. (One person who had been a committee member as long as the agency has been in existence recalled that such packages could amount to 700 pages per project.) With the funding cuts that had come within the last few years, the agency cut costs by reducing the amount of material mailed to each person. Funding cuts also meant a reduction in the clerical staff available to manage this task. At the same time, the professional staff members who remained had accumulated several years of experience. The result of this combination of factors was a "streamlined" mailing to the committee members. The response to the streamlining was mixed.

During the interview, all of the respondents discussed the role of the staff. Virtually everyone began this portion of the discussion by praising the staff for working hard, after which they revealed varying degrees of reservation about the role played by the staff. The comments made by providers questioned staff members' competence to comment on various technical matters from medical services through legal or financial aspects of proposed projects. One member with a finance background complained that staff members thought they could simply read a few paragraphs in an accounting text and set themselves up as experts. How they explained the financial portion of a proposal currently under review according to this person was "all nonsense. But I didn't say anything because no one was listening; if they would have listened, they wouldn't have understood it; and they weren't going to do anything about it anyway." He suggested that having consultants with specific kinds of expertise would resolve such problems. He pointed out that this had been the idea originally before the funding cuts prohibited such considerations.

The reactions of the consumers to the staff's role were more complicated. While some consumers praised the streamlining efforts of the staff, a few complained that there was still too much to read. There were others who indicated that they recognized and resented the staff's attempts to manipulate them. It is interesting that more than a few consumer representatives stated that they preferred to hear the arguments presented by proponents and opponents of proposals on the committee rather than accept the staff's determinations at face value. They made clear that *they* were the committee members; that it was up to *them* to make the final decision; and, the *staff* was after all the *staff*. After outlining their objections to what they perceived to be staff efforts to manipulate them, four consumer representatives announced with a spontaneous burst of emotion: "I am not a rubber stamp!"

Obviously, this points to a sensitive structural problem. Lacking other sources of information and networks providing insights or help to formulate a stance with regard to certain proposals, the consumers had no place else to turn for assistance except the staff. Such dependency produced a sense of indebtedness as well as resentment. The consumer representatives could not easily develop an opposing argument, even if they were motivated to do so, when they were provided with a summary statement written by the staff in support of a particular evaluative stance. The consumers could always return to the original documents, supporting materials and file of correspondence between the staff and the institutions proposing the project, all of which are available in the office. This, however, would be a burdensome task and still would not overcome the lack of an alternative network to assist in developing an independent interpretation. Of course, this description does not apply to those consumers who represent a particular constituency or are employed by an organization representing vested consumer interests. The fact of the matter is, however, that more than half of the consumer representatives at the Urban HSA did not have such organizational ties or networks.

STRUCTURAL DIFFERENCES IN INVOLVEMENT

There are a number of other structural differences between the participation of consumers and providers. First, consumers must rely on personal opinion or staff interpretation, while providers often have access to research departments which provide analyses of relevant issues. Second, the communities providers represent are organized, interested, and informed, while the communities consumers represent are typically not readily identifiable, only tangentially interested, and generally poorly informed. Third, the time invested by providers is "company" time, while consumers must use personal time. The time spent on HSA business is a cost to consumers, possibly in foregone income or opportunity for career advancement. By contrast, when providers invest time in the HSA, they can generally count on some work-related rewards.

The government considered a number of measures in writing the 1979 amendments that might have overcome the structural imbalance inherent in consumer participation as opposed to provider participation. Paying consumers for their time was considered. However, this led to discussions on measuring exactly how much income consumers were really losing. Ultimately the idea was abandoned as overly cumbersome and potentially demeaning to consumers. The solution the government decided to recommend was suggesting that a staff member be assigned to assist consumers. As I have indicated, this relationship had its own problems. Since a staff member was assigned to each committee and presumably was available to both consumers and providers at the Urban HSA, the arrangement was not altered in response to the 1979 amendments in the prevailing planning legislation (PL 93–641).

CONCLUSION

The evaluation of the Urban HSA's success by consumers is different from that of providers because the expectations they brought to this effort are different; their experiences with health care institutions and arrangements are dissimilar; and, finally, the directions in which consumers would prefer the HSA to move are not the same as those favored by providers. In sum, this suggests that the manner in which providers and consumers experience their participation is qualitatively different.

Consumers seem to be most concerned with public involvement of various sorts. Public education is a high priority; not only education about general health care, but about availability of services and the opportunity to voice opinions and complaints with regard to the services that are available. This is precisely the kind of activity they collectively point to as a reason to be satisfied with the HSA's performance; and it is one to which they want the HSA to devote more attention.

The providers, by contrast, seem to be more concerned about HSA activities which could contribute to a broader planning agenda. While the state's ability to reject the HSA's decisions is a source of frustration to both consumers and providers, the federal regulations and guidelines do not appear to be as problematic to the consumers as they are to the providers. The providers also are more concerned about having adequate data to make judgments and having a workable health plan to use as a guide for making decisions.

To distill the differences one more degree, the consumers and providers are generally in agreement about the manifest goals outlined in PL 93–641. However, they seem to think along different lines about the best way to reach those goals. For their part, the consumers are definitive about their desire to invite citizen participation in the health planning process by making available for public screening institutional plans for expansion or change. This is treated as a positive outcome in and of itself. Accordingly, because the public now has a platform for voicing concerns about health care delivery, the consumers are expressing a certain amount of satisfaction with this achievement. Their goal has been met in part. The providers, by contrast, have less to be satisfied about because the goal, as they have interpreted it, is more abstract and far-reaching. At minimum, the goal envisioned by the providers requires that everyone involved reach a consensus with regard to the objectives stated in the Health Systems Plan (HSP) and the Annual Implementation Plan (AIP). Moreover, in order for the committee review process to operate within a common framework of understanding, everyone involved must also concur with regard to the means selected to reach those objectives. This has not happened. While the consumers generally had little to say about the HSP or the AIP, more than a few of the providers were actively opposed to the design of the plans as they were shaping up:

There's been lots of dreaming in the HSP. They say by a certain date the incidence of alcoholism should be reduced by X amount. These numbers are arrived at out of the air. I'm not happy with the goals. There are real defects in the reasoning.

Another provider who would like the HSA to have a good deal more authority stated that under present circumstances:

They're planning in a vacuum. . . . They can blow out a candle, but they couldn't affect the frosting, much less the cake.

I have argued that consumers and providers have somewhat different objectives, would prefer to use different means, and generally experience the work of the HSA differently. At this point, I would like to return to the consumer I mentioned earlier who claimed that he now knew what "CAP scanners" were. Obviously, he is not very convincing on this point. Let us consider the quality of the input that can be expected from him. In the course of our discussion, he explained that there was a dire need for an alcoholism treatment center and alcoholism beds in his community. He was also actively engaged in arranging to have health science training programs established to prepare people for entry-level jobs in the health sector. He had a number of other practical ideas for improving conditions in his community. He felt that joining the HSA was advantageous because it helped him to understand better how the health system worked, so he could be more effective in achieving his objectives. There is no question that he expected to attain those objectives. In short, he is dedicated to his community and has a firm conception of its needs. "High tech" medicine and CAT scanners are far too distant from his agenda for him to invest much energy to educate himself about them. It is difficult, however, to dismiss him as incapable of making informed decisions. Rather than dismissing this man's ideas and his contributions to planning, perhaps the area of decision making should be realigned so that the issues of greatest concern to communities and topics about which people are in fact reasonably well informed might be given greater attention.

One of the experiences recounted by the Urban HSA staff members provides additional support for this point. A complaint often voiced by HSA participants and health planning evaluators is that it is difficult to get the public involved in the planning process. The public simply does not show much interest. A variety of schemes are periodically recommended in the effort to educate the public based on the assumption that educational programs will stimulate greater public interest. Public meetings scheduled by the Urban HSA, similarly, rarely attract anyone other than HSA staff and the representatives of the institution whose proposal is being presented to the community. The major exception occurred a year or so before I began working with the HSA. The public hearing on a proposal that would have created an abortion clinic in the center of a predominantly Catholic community attracted approximately 250 people there to protest the plan. Approval was denied on this basis. Observers of the health care system who claim that the public will become involved when it is ready to do so apparently are right.

A contrast to the consumer whose understanding of CAT scanners is in doubt is the position taken by a particularly dedicated and experienced provider. This person presented a well-thought-out assessment of the problems poor people were having obtaining health care; of the difficulties hospitals were having meeting the needs of the poor while trying to maintain their competitive edge by investing in new technology; and of the legal, moral, and financial complexities facing the health care system currently. After such an analysis there was nothing else that could be said except that the system was overwhelmingly complex and too entrenched to expect much change to occur as a result of health planning, at least not in its present form. The point is that while this provider seems to be very knowledgeable about how the health care system operates, she is discouraged about the prospects of change because the changes she thinks are necessary are system changes. The consumer who claims to understand CAT scanners wants changes in his community involving one or two community hospitals. It is no wonder that the consumer expects to accomplish his objectives while the provider expects little change to occur. Admittedly the contrast provided by these two individuals illustrates the extreme case. However, this illustration also captures the essence of the difference between the expectations that the consumer representatives, as opposed to the provider representatives, brought to the planning process at the Urban HSA.

7

The Emergence of Groups

A review of the process-oriented literature shows that a high level of consensus regarding the assessment that one of the major obstacles to attaining greater success in health planning was the dominance providers were exerting over consumers. The solutions recommended in this literature revolved around mechanisms to enhance consumer participation. In fact, the 1979 amendments to PL 93–641 advocated a number of measures which were designed to do exactly that. The amendments recommended selecting consumer representatives to speak for identifiable interest groups, including certain social, ethnic, economic, geographic, and disabled communities. These correctives were expected to improve representation by making the individual consumer representatives accountable to a specific group of consumers with a vested interest. However, no one who has studied health planning from a process-oriented perspective has ventured to say that health planning agencies performed any better after the 1979 amendment was legislated. The outcome-oriented researchers, who found that greater cost savings had been attained as a result of health planning than earlier research had indicated, have also given us little reason to think that improved consumer representation was responsible. In any case, the recent reversal in findings regarding the relationship between health planning and cost containment has had surprisingly little impact on the thinking exhibited in the process-oriented branch of the literature with regard to the role played by providers. The assumptions contributing to the formulation of the 1974 planning act have remained intact. The basic assumption that providers are self-interested and single-minded in their determination to resist all efforts to control the expansion of the health care sector apparently has become so firmly rooted in the thinking of those who observe the process of planning that there has been no sense of need to verify it. A related assumption that providers would be consistent in their support for all proposals to expand health care facilities or services has become similarly entrenched. Indeed, this portrayal of provider motivations has been treated as an established fact over the last decade. Discussions often begin with reference to this "fact" before going on to consider solutions. (In fairness there have been a number of observations contradicting this image of providers; however, they have not attracted much attention [Bicknell and Walsh 1975].)

The consumers, by contrast, were expected to represent the public interest, which in this case means that they were expected to halt the continuing expansion of the health care sector by not allowing institutions to expend funds on "unnecessary" capital investments. While the portrayal of consumers has not been nearly as explicit as that of providers, the imagery found in the literature suggests that consumers were viewed as being pure of heart and interested only in working for the public good and that they were not nearly as effective as hoped because they were foiled in their efforts by the overpowering, self-serving providers. If this assessment seems excessive, consider the fact that consumer motivations have never been questioned, even though consumers often failed to oppose proposals presented by institutions which outlined plans to expand. Instead, providers consistently have been blamed for persuading the consumers to stray from what have been assumed to be their true intentions.

In short, the portrayal of persons involved in health planning has been extreme. First, both categories of participants were assigned unrealistic roles. Second, the reaction to the failure of consumers to behave as expected was disappointment rather than an attempt to reexamine assumptions regarding the assigned roles. (See Brown 1982 for a more recent analysis of the roles assigned to consumer representatives.) Third, there is no question that the consumers were positioned, by the health planning act of 1974, to function at the vanguard in the battle against rising health care costs, a battle staged on a base of simplistic assumptions about the psychological motivations of two highly diverse categories of individuals. Fourth, people were assigned to one of two categories, the consumer or provider categories, even though the credentials of some made such designations arbitrary. Finally, in sociological terms, individuals were aggregated, that is, assigned, to a category on the basis of a characteristic those doing the assigning used to distinguish one individual from another. Once assigned, they were expected to behave as if they belonged to a "group." (I will elaborate on the meaning that sociologists attach to the concept of "group" in the context of presenting my observations on the work that was being carried out at the Urban HSA during the time I spent there.)

THE URBAN HSA PARTICIPANTS

At the outset of this discussion, I offer two central observations: first, on the whole, the consumer representatives at the Urban HSA did not resist or oppose the decision making outcomes advocated by the providers; and, second, domination of consumers by providers was uncommon. I will retrace my steps in carrying out this study in order to show how I arrived at these two seemingly contradictory findings.

I began by asking everyone I interviewed two opening questions: how did you happen to become involved with the Urban HSA?, and do you feel you represent a particular constituency? I admit, I began with these two questions because I thought that they would put the respondents at ease by providing them with an opportunity to present themselves as they wished to be perceived. I made this decision in response to evidence indicating that interviewees engage in what survey researchers call "impression management" (DeSantis 1980). I was also interested in presenting myself in the way I wanted to be perceived—as a non-critical listener. In the end, I planned to discount this portion of the interview as a necessary introductory discussion but not essential to the data collection part of the interview. To my surprise, the first question created a problem for a certain number of people who were not sure why they were invited to work with the HSA. Two people were put in the position of having to admit that they got there by applying pressure on local political influentials. There were others who were very clear about their qualifications and their appointments. They outlined their previous experience in related kinds of activities as well as current organizational affiliations to which their appointments were connected.

In response to my second question, many respondents, both providers and consumers, said they represented themselves in making decisions. Some indicated that while they had certain reference groups aiding them in determining how they would vote, they did not feel rigidly bound by those ties to take the position that benefited their respective constituencies on all occasions. Some respondents reflected a greater degree of concern about their roles and their responsibilities than others, as one consumer representative's recollections of the ceremonies on the day she was appointed illustrate:

It was never clear, when I was first appointed, why I was appointed. We all talked to [the local dignitaries] then. I was one of the last in the group when they were asking where we were from, most people were telling about where they lived. Later, when we were all talking together, we were talking about where we worked. I didn't know if I was supposed to be representing my community, or women between the ages of 18 and 35, or Blacks, or the people I work for. . . . When I had to make a vote, sometimes these things complicated it. So I voted for myself. The other day, we were told [by the staff] we can represent the community.

IDENTITY AND MISSION OF THE PARTICIPANTS

None of the doctors and hospital administrators had any problem explaining exactly why they had become involved with the HSA. The doctors began by stating how their medical background was related to their interest in the HSA, for example, because of a public health background, administrative position in a medical school, or role in the local medical society. Both doctors and administrators spoke about protecting the interests of the community in which the institution with which they were affiliated was located. Other providers—nurses, therapists, and social workers—did not express a similarly strong sense of commitment to the institutions in which they worked, nor did their respective occupational identities seem to supply them with as clear-cut a stance vis à vis the HSA's activities as that expressed by the doctors or the hospital administrators. It should be noted that providers who were not physicians or administrators were, according to the literature, expected to side with the consumers in opposing the expansionist tendencies of providers (Checkoway, O'Rourke, and Macrina 1981). This expectation was not fulfilled at the Urban HSA because the expected clean-cut split between the provider position and the consumer position did not develop. The alliances which did evolve were considerably more complex. Actually, the process of coalition formation can be attributed, to a large extent, to a handful of especially aggressive consumers.

Of all the participants, the community activists were the most direct in explaining their mission in working with the Urban HSA. They were forthright about stating that they were interested in protecting and advancing, whenever possible, the interests of the respective communities they represented. The reason they could take such a partisan stance without fear of being perceived as self-interested or biased is that they represented communities that were clearly "underserved" (had fewer health care resources, that is, hospital beds or the various services that hospitals provide). Another point is relevant to their respective identities and stated purposes—the fact that ethnicity and race are closely tied to geographic community. In other words, the community activists were representing underserved racial or ethnic groups in particular geographic communities.

The consumer representatives who were neither community activists nor representatives of a consumer-interest organization were the ones who had the most difficulty explaining who they represented and how they could best meet their HSA responsibilities. People in this category also had to rely on others for help in exploring the issues presented by the proposals being put before them. Some chose to join informal caucus groups; others depended on staff for information; a few people put their trust in another individual and went along with that person's decisions.

The variation in the answers I received to the two questions led me to look more closely at the process of coalition formation. Although it quickly became clear that the assessments about the decision-making process were not following the lines I was led to anticipate by the literature, initially I could not understand why this was the case. It was only in the course of observing for some months the interaction patterns exhibited by the participants that I found what I believe may be a critical flaw in the thinking responsible for the design of health planning legislation as well as the additional correctives discussed in the literature. The participants, once assigned to categories, were expected to turn themselves into two distinct groups, composed entirely of consumers or providers. However, these two categories remained "aggregates" rather than becoming "groups." In sociological terms, an aggregate is a classification encompassing individuals who happen to share some characteristic that they may or may not consider important to their identity, for example, living in a single-person household, falling between the ages of twenty and twenty-four, having arthritis, or such. Belonging to a group is a very different phenomenon. For sociological purposes, a group includes people who have a sense of belonging, are aware of specific shared characteristics, recognize the boundaries which distinguish those who belong from those who do not, and so on. To illustrate, newspapers occasionally report on events which produced a "group" but occurred under unusual circumstances, for example: jurors who have been together through a lengthy trial arranging to meet for a picnic sometime later or a busload of strangers who, when interviewed, talk about the fun they had together while stranded during a snowstorm in a neighborhood bar. The sociological literature also reports in detail on the emergence of characteristics that produce a strong sense of unity under somewhat more conventional circumstances, for example, in medical school, in religious cults, in boot camp. Such a scenario was not played out by either the consumer or provider categories at the Urban HSA.

COALITION FORMATION

The providers did not form a coalition for a number of reasons. First, given the widespread sense that HSAs were there to impose controls on a health industry that was out of control, the doctors and hospital administrators were keeping a low profile. Second, they had no reason to object on a collective basis to the coalition formation process that had developed. Finally, they had their own reasons for keeping their distance from one another. While they, and the institutions with which they were affiliated, had a fairly clear set of shared interests to protect, they were also competitors.

One provider, who held an administrative position but who was not trained in any of the health occupations, pointed out that the providers could never trust one another completely. She recounted her experiences in working with a local American Heart Association committee created to write a group proposal for a multimillion-dollar heart disease research grant being awarded by the federal government. A number of high status institutions came together to write the proposal with the understanding that grants were being awarded one to a region. All of the representatives agreed that their best chance was to produce a single document rather than to compete with one another. In the end, one of the participating institutions secretly submitted its own proposal and carried on a sub-rosa lobbying effort via a network of personal friendships in Washington. Naturally everyone eventually found out about this maneuver. The individual who described this incident ended by saying that providers could not form alliances because such patterns of behavior were the rule, not the exception.

Another reason that all the providers did not form a single group is that the providers who are not doctors or hospital administrators are not usually treated by anyone, including themselves, as if they belong in the same circles as those who are doctors and administrators. They did not act as if they belonged in the same group in this case either.

If the providers could not find common grounds for group formation at the Urban HSA, it is difficult to imagine the grounds on which the consumers could unite. The consumers, after all, shared only one common trait—they were not providers. Theirs is a residual category with none of the characteristics that might promote a group identity. It is true that they were expected to share a common sense of purpose with regard to the work of the HSA. However, this shared sense of purpose is an abstract idea that did not survive very well differences of opinion regarding implementation.

By contrast, as indicated earlier, the consumer representatives who were community activists were not only certain of their respective constituencies but were prepared to argue aggressively on their behalf. As a result, they were influential in establishing the racial/ethnic/geographic community-interest dimension as the predominant perspective from which to consider projects under review. A number of other factors contributed to making this a central point of departure in the decision-making process. For one, there were no competing frameworks being promoted. The providers had no reason to oppose this approach. None of the representatives of other identifiable constituencies such as the elderly, the handicapped, or organized labor objected because the approach posed no real threat to their objectives. Moreover, they could not have advanced their individual agendas to supersede this more general one even if they had wanted to do so. The staff also gave its tacit support to this development, in part, because it was being recommended in the federal guidelines; more importantly, it was consistent with one of the staff's primary objectives, which was to have an impact on the maldistribution of facilities in the area.

The emergence of the race/ethnicity/geographic location dimension as a source of group identity had two effects, which are not very surprising, plus one major unanticipated effect which I will discuss in greater detail. The predictable effects on the decision-making framework were, first, the groups which did emerge minimized the significance of the provider-consumer boundary. Second, the emergence of "community" as a source of group identity redefined the main objective, to some extent, by directing greater attention to the redistribution of facilities and services rather than to cost containment.

The emergence of a group, based on the community dimension as it evolved at the Urban HSA, was most clearly demonstrated in the case of the Latino coalition. The Latino members of the HSA were primarily consumer representatives, many without any previous experience in the health care sector. The explanation offered by one Latino community activist for his rising level of interest in HSA activities makes clear why the Latino coalition evolved as it did:

It was about six or seven months before I really started reading the stuff they were sending me. There was a lot to read. I wasn't really interested. I just agreed to be on it [the HSA] like a lot of other committees I'm on. I didn't know what it was about, then I began to understand more, as HSA participants we didn't have a lot of power, but if we all acted to oppose construction or modernization we could try to control and tell the hospitals what they can do.

As their collective awareness of their potential power increased, the Latino participants from different neighborhoods were also becoming better acquainted with one another. They derived power from their shared recognition of the fact that they could not assure passage of a project, but by voting as a block they could stop passage if they chose to do so. In order to enhance their collective base of power, they also tried to recruit other participants to take their side. According to one person:

They [the Latinos] were fighting for more services, so that anything that came by, they approved. If you didn't go along, they glared at you.

The Latino coalition's willingness to take an aggressive stance on behalf of its constituents was sufficiently disruptive to force the agency to take special measures to address the problem. A special study was launched to determine the health profile and health needs of Latinos in the area. In the end, everyone was pleased with the document that was produced, and the HSA's activities returned to a less polarized state.

While the tactics used by the Latinos may have been perceived as strident by a few of their fellow committee members, no one argued that their demands were in any way inconsistent with the agency's purpose. Perhaps they were perceived as especially aggressive because their actions were in such sharp contrast to the stance taken by Blacks at the Urban HSA. It was quite clear why Blacks, some of whom formed an informal caucus group of their own, did not behave in an equally aggressive manner. The fact that Blacks are underserved is accepted as an unquestionable fact in the country as a whole and in the Urban HSA in particular. Blacks did not need to make assertions about something that was an accepted fact. Furthermore, this was a situation that everyone involved with the HSA appeared to be interested in correcting. There was also no way to avoid the fact that Blacks were underserved since the community maps used by the staff as visual aids in considering proposed projects graphically confirmed the inequity in the distribution of beds, particular services, and any other criterion being used in cross-community comparisons. Finally, it may have made a difference to Black participants to find that Blacks held important staff positions in the agency. The one drawback of this situation from the perspective of Black community activists was that this atmosphere did not provide much support for the emergence of a more aggressive Black caucus, which a few of the community activists were still interested in promoting.

Since the HSA participants were aware of the maldistribution of health care resources in the area and in agreement about the need to correct the problem, this point of consensus provided a unifying focus for HSA activities. It permitted everyone to share in a sense of common purpose when all those present agreed to approve proposals promising to improve the health services available to the underserved. The good feeling that surrounded such occasions was one of few sources of reward the participants could look forward to enjoying.

THE COST CONTAINMENT GOAL

The other major legislative goal, controlling rising costs, did not produce a similar sense of unity or satisfaction because the means to achieve it were much less tangible. Approving the development of additional resources is far more concrete in its promised results than the result that the denial of expansion could produce. In fact, achieving savings was not something many thought the HSA was equipped to do because the purse strings were in the hands of third-party payers, politicians in Washington, large corporations, and so on. One physician member who thought that the cost of health care was the single most important problem confronting the health care system was extremely discouraged about achieving any savings because he felt that the reasons behind high costs were too complex for the HSA to address. He used the following example to illustrate his point:

How the system works is—you ask for a catheter. You need a two-dollar tube. You get eighteen dollars worth of equipment that you don't need. It comes in a sealed package to keep it sterile; and, you end up throwing sixteen dollars away.

Another provider sums up the attitude of most providers:

It's political; it's financial. Those who have clout, whatever means they have available, tend to ride over everything and get their projects across at the expense of others. I don't know how this can be overcome.

Most providers pointed out the flaws in "the law" and, with that, dismissed the possibility that the HSA could have any influence on costs.

If CON [Certificate of Need review] has not contained costs, it has something to do with the law. There was no ceiling on costs. Reviewing each project separately is no way to contain costs. There should be restraint on the total amount of expenditures.

Then the same person added the following comment, shedding light on yet another dimension to the problem of containing costs:

The big guys come in with power tactics. The little guys come in with heartrending stories. It's hard to say no.

While the providers seem to be overwhelmed by the complexity of the problem of rising costs, the consumers treated this matter with considerably more confidence than the providers. They generally were much more willing to take up the challenge posed by rising costs. A number of consumer comments will illustrate the difference:

—Hospitals are ripping off ignorant people.

—Hospitals will run away with costs if we don't stop them.

—There should be more authority for regulation.

—If people got together, they could do something. This is a place where we can do something.

—If forced, institutions will allow themselves to be regulated.

The consumers generally advocated the elimination of unnecessary services, inefficiency, and waste. However, no one seemed certain which services were unnecessary and exactly how to go about eliminating waste and inefficiency. To make matters more complicated, the services operating at a marginal level were invariably in hospitals located in poor and underserved areas. Disapproving proposals to expand services which might bring in additional patients to such institutions was tantamount to condemning them to closure, thereby further depleting services in an already poorly served area. This dilemma was discussed each time these circumstances presented themselves without much progress toward a satisfactory solution.

THE COMMUNITY INTEREST AGENDA

Clearly there were a number of good reasons to explain why approving proposals which would bring needed services to underserved communities emerged as an activity that was given especially high priority in the Urban HSA. It is also easy to understand why the cost containment goal was relegated to second place. What is far more difficult to explain is the willingness of the HSA participants to approve proposals for expanding health care services and facilities in communities that were clearly "over-served." Perhaps the continued emphasis on "community" needs sensitized everyone to the potential benefits that might accrue to the community. This is not to say that anyone disputed the fact that communities with an abundance of health care resources did not need more health care facilities and services. However, the participants were also not willing to close their eyes to the fact that bringing in such health care resources could benefit the community in other ways.

Consider the following account involving a project proposed for a community generally recognized to be the singularly most over-served community in the entire urban HSA area. The project in question came up for review in the spring of 1983 after months of discussion with the HSA staff. The proposal outlined a

300–plus-bed nursing home and apartment complex for the elderly. The organization applying for CON approval took certain steps before initiating the first contact with the HSA staff to request an informal meeting to discuss the project. The spokesmen for the organization hired a major consulting firm, where a former highly influential member of the HSA board had accepted a position. They contacted the governor of the state, the mayor, various local politicians, plus the community groups in the area, all of whom agreed to support the project in writing. They had already purchased an old, abandoned warehouse situated on the edge of the community, which had successfully been pursuing a program of "gentrification" (middle-class takeover of a rundown neighborhood) over the last decade. The organization obtained an historical-landmark designation for the building, which was not only a status advantage but made a low interest government loan available. It quickly became clear to the HSA staff that the nursing home group had not overlooked any opportunity to garner support for the project. However, there was no justification for adding beds in this community. The nursing home spokesmen were not about to be discouraged. When the project came up for review by the HSA, they invited community representatives and local politicians to speak on their behalf.

The meeting proceeded as follows. First, the negative staff report was read and the nursing home representatives responded point by point. In response to the assessment that the area had an excess of beds, a nursing home representative argued that nursing home beds were needed precisely because there were so many hospitals in the area. The staff countered by saying that it was not the location of the hospitals that was the critical factor but the proximity of the nursing home beds to patients' homes. Furthermore, there was a critical shortage of nursing home beds in adjacent communities, while this community had an excess. The nursing home spokesmen pointed out that the proposed location offered easy access to major traffic arteries and public transportation lines. This portion of the discussion was treated as a matter of clarification of relevant evaluation criteria found in the health planning guidelines handed down by the federal government. Before opening the discussion to a more general question and answer session, the chair invited the well-known local politician who represents the area and the community organization representatives to speak. The contrast between their statements and the preceding discussion is striking.

The politician, who maintained a high public profile and was politically independent, spoke with some fervor about how highly the community valued the project for its effect on community property values, beautification, safety and opportunities for employment. Each of the five well-appointed gentlemen who spoke on behalf of the five neighborhood organizations echoed the same sentiments. Conspicuous in its absence was any mention of the effect the project might have on health care costs or access to health care services. I could not establish what, if any, discussions went on between these speakers and the nursing home group prior to this meeting. It is clear, however, that the speakers were considering the project from a perspective which had little to do with the entire reason for the existence of the HSA.

When the committee took up the discussion, a committee member who was also a resident of the area shifted the focus of the discussion back to health care issues. He pointed out that there were many elderly persons in the area who would benefit. He also noted that the presence of the nursing home could encourage doctors to discharge patients sooner, which would produce cost savings. One of the more strident community activists who represented an adjacent area with a serious shortage of nursing home beds argued strongly against the project. Three or four other persons commented on the location as well. The last person to speak may have summed up the feelings of the other participants by making the pragmatic observation that the nursing home group had obviously carefully prepared its proposal and thought through the arguments against it and that it had a good record and adequate financial backing. Since the city did need more nursing home beds and no one else was proposing to build any, the project should be approved. The majority of the participants who were present voted in favor of the project. The same scenario was repeated a week later, when the executive board voted in favor of the project as well. The state board approved it shortly thereafter. I should add that neither the HSA committee meeting nor the board meeting during which this project was reviewed attracted the full complement of persons who were serving on either the committee or executive board. It is possible that some saw the vote as a foregone conclusion. It is also possible that the participants were feeling generally discouraged about entering into this battle after losing other battles they had recently tried to wage. (A rather heated battle had been lost a few months before this proposal came up for review; I will outline that case in the following chapter.) Perhaps some did not attend because they were simply not interested in proposals outlining the expansion of nursing home beds as opposed to hospital beds. The fact remains that there was no identifiable category of persons willing to oppose this project.

This case is provocative from a number of perspectives. To begin with, it raises questions about the views held by the public at large. The community organization spokesmen, for example, were presumably well-informed, concerned, and reasonably intelligent citizens. They based their statements in support of the nursing home on what they apparently thought were convincing arguments reflecting shared concerns. Why they chose to tie their support for the nursing home to the views they did, rather than the agency's stated purpose, is an interesting question to ponder. I assume that the nursing home representatives, whose approach was obviously very well planned, could have coached the community organization spokesmen but chose not to do so. The nursing home group had the assistance of a consultant who could have suggested that the community organization spokesmen touch on cost containment or access issues but chose not to do so.

Another question this case raises relates to the vote. How can a positive vote in this case be interpreted, when it occurred in spite of a staff evaluation stating that approval of the project would violate the intent of the law, the federal guidelines, the agency's own health plans, in other words, everything? Is it possible that the political pressure from the governor on down so impressed the HSA participants that they could not resist the pressure? This may have played some part. I suspect, however, that the nursing home representatives were making a calculated appeal intentionally touching on the kinds of issues that are of basic interest to most people, in fact, more basic than the abstract aims with which the HSA usually deals; it worked!

The only other time (during my twenty-month stay) that a community spokesman came to an HSA meeting to speak on behalf of the community's interest in the project being considered was when a hospital proposed to turn a large number of acute case beds into teenage drug rehabilitation and psychiatric beds. The political boundaries of the neighborhood involved produced a community composed of a strip of expensive condominiums alongside a strip of run-down, low-rise apartment buildings together with a seedy commercial district. The run-down portion accommodated a number of halfway houses and cheap housing for a large proportion of the city's transient population. The spokesman, a local politician, claimed that the middle class residents were afraid the hospital's new program would bring more potentially disruptive people to the area. The second point of argument was that the hospital was already an unwelcome entity in the community because of the parking problems it was creating. The staff assessment indicated that the beds were not needed in the community according to the official guidelines, which would have provided a firm basis for the community's case. Again, the community spokesman chose not to cast the argument in this light. Instead, she chose to employ more mundane and universal concerns on which to base her case, such as parking congestion and concern about the presence of undesirable types in the community.

CONCLUSION

To sum up, the first and most significant observation discussed in this chapter is the fact that the Urban HSA participants did not organize themselves into two separate groups reflecting a provider-consumer split, which is what much of the health planning literature led me to expect. The literature also prepared me to expect that these designations would be predictive of decision-making behavior. In other words, the authors of PL 93–641 were modeling the decision-making structure being handed to HSAs to reflect the natural course that the perceived split between consumers and providers was expected to take. In this case, a traditional two-party decision-making structure did not provide a suitable fit. In actuality, the individuals in both categories brought such varied backgrounds, experiences, and values to the process that there was little chance that either those in the consumer category or those in the provider category would evolve into a "group." In the case of the Urban HSA, these two categories might more accurately be described as "aggregates" rather than "groups;" since persons who belong to a "group," in sociological terms, must have a sense of shared values, feelings of belonging, and an understanding of the boundaries indicating who belongs and who does not. Groups with such characteristics did emerge, but they emerged along a dimension other than the predicted consumer-provider split.

Groups formed around a "community focus," combining the racial, ethnic, and geographic dimensions of community. The consumers who were community activists succeeded in advancing these factors as the primary considerations in evaluating proposals. Since others were not interested in promoting alternative frameworks, this approach prevailed. It was not contested for another important reason; it was consistent with the effort to identify underserved communities and bring added services or facilities to them. Finally, the emergence of consensus on the importance of this agenda permitted all HSA participants to enjoy a sense of unity and purposefulness in approving proposals that would benefit the underserved, a reward which decisions based on other criteria did not provide.

Thus, upgrading health care resources in underserved areas increased in salience while the cost containment goal moved into second place. This occurred in spite of the fact that everyone seemed to agree that cost containment was the primary problem. Enthusiasm for containing health care costs was also difficult to sustain, largely because many participants saw little hope of having much impact on this front. The reasons given, generally by providers, included the conviction that the HSA was not equipped to attain this objective; that the causes of rising costs were outside the control of the HSA; that the large institutions would use power tactics and get their way in any case; and that applying strict rules to smaller, struggling institutions posed a dilemma, especially if they were located in underserved areas. While the consumers were generally less discouraged than the providers about the prospects of controlling rising costs, they also seemed to be less certain about how this objective was to be attained.

The focus on racial/ethnic/geographic community was responsible for the emergence of the two groups that could be identified. The more active of the two groups that evolved was the Latino caucus. While most of those involved in this group were consumers, Latino providers were also actively involved. A Black caucus emerged as well, also drawing from both the provider and consumer categories. However, it operated on a more informal basis. Unlike the Latino group, the Black caucus did not develop a set of demands or a position paper. In large part, this was because the needs of the Black poor in the area were so obviously urgent, there was no need to press the point. By contrast, very little was known about the health care needs of the Latinos in the area.

The manifest agenda of the Urban HSA was greatly affected by the emergence of the community dimension as a dominant focus of discussion and decision making. The emphasis given to this perspective had several effects: first, diminishing the importance of the consumer-provider distinction; second, displacing cost containment as a primary priority in favor of upgrading health care resources in underserved communities; in contrast to the first two, the third effect was totally unexpected. The emphasis on community served to heighten everyone's identification with his own community. Depending on the individual, this could either be the community of residence or the community in which the institution to which the person was attached through work was located. The heightened sense of identification with community had a striking latent effect.

Proposals to expand services and facilities in resource-rich communities, while rare, were not quickly rejected, which is certainly what the rhetoric of the HSA participants would lead one to expect. Instead, the argument employed on such occasions turned out to be considerably more pragmatic—if no one else is proposing such a project and the institution proposing it looks like it will do a good job, we might as well let it go ahead rather than wait until the right institution proposes a project in the right place. In spite of the rhetoric regarding the importance of cost containment, this pragmatic point of view is not particularly surprising. Much more interesting to consider are the attitudes expressed by the HSA representatives from resource-rich communities. They said something closer to the following: the people proposing such projects seem to know what they're doing; there is a need for such services in the area if not exactly in this community; and, finally, if the money is spent here it will have some benefits which I don't want to give up. In short, a perceptible shift in stakes was apparent on such occasions, the issue being—I want my share, too.

The advantages inherent in adding new facilities, new services or modernizing old ones were very clearly addressed by the politicians and community organization spokesmen on the small number of occasions they came to HSA meetings to present the neighborhood's position on a particular proposal. They spoke about property values, safety, beautification, parking, new jobs, and so on. It is important to consider that not all participants faced a conflict on such occasions between what they said was important and their decision-making behavior. Certainly the community activists had no conflict, nor did the providers who had powerful attachments to institutions in underserved communities. Since the high status providers were in a position to participate in organizing the delivery of services in their respective institutions, it is unlikely that they had much internal conflict about arguing that their respective institutions were serving the community well and deserved all the help they could get in continuing their work. It was the participants who were attempting to respond in terms of the public good instead of responding in terms of a commitment to their own communities who were faced with difficult choices. Thus, on occasion, more concrete community concerns which were not organized around health care needs could be observed to be winning out in the decisions being made at the Urban HSA over concern about the public good. The question this raises is: Are those who appear to be consistent in their rhetoric and their decision-making behavior in arguing for better health care resources for their respective communities really fighting for health care resources or are they interested in gaining resources of whatever kind happen to be at stake? By the same token, is it reasonable to expect HSA participants to reject a project intended for their respective communities if it promises various economic and social advantages? It is even more difficult to imagine rejecting a proposal when it is clear who will lose as a consequence, namely, one's own community, but not at all clear who will benefit. Finally, given a fairly high level of discouragement regarding cost containment efforts, the belief that costs were bound to go up anyway, so why should some other community benefit while ''we'' sacrifice ourselves, was a sentiment that never seemed to be very far beneath the surface.

8

The "Teeth" in the Law
That Didn't Work

Thus far I have discussed the Urban HSA's accomplishments from the point of view of the participants. However, I have not ventured to take a position on whether the HSA was, in fact, successful in its endeavors. The answer depends on one's level of expectation. This was illustrated by the fact that the providers interviewed were less satisfied than the consumers because the changes they had hoped the HSA would produce were far more extensive than the changes the consumers had in mind. The answer also requires that the measure of success be specified. In reviewing the literature, I pointed out that the reports employing sophisticated, quantitative evaluation techniques use health care cost or capital expenditure trends to determine the degree of success or failure of the planning agencies in the area (usually the state). The other major branch of the health planning literature, which focuses on participation in the decision-making process, does not identify a concrete measure of success.

The discussion evaluating the Urban HSA's performance focuses on the three goals stated in the Health Planning and Development Act, which was responsible for creating HSAs: (1) the Urban HSA's success in controlling health care costs and/or expenditures; (2) its success in ensuring that all people in the area have access to health care services: and (3) its success in affecting positively the quality of care in the area. In sum, I intend to consider the performance of the HSA with respect to each of the goals mentioned and in doing so focus on the reasons why an accurate evaluation is so difficult to produce.

1. According to its own periodic reports, the Urban HSA's cost containment record is reasonably impressive. A number of possible interpretations might be considered to explain its success. The evaluation research literature suggests the following possibilities: the staff became more experienced and more confident in processing proposals over time; the HSA committee members became more

experienced as well; another explanation which is suggested, but which has gone unstated, is that the consumers became more resistant to provider domination; the cycle of pent-up demand in anticipation of CON controls was played out by the early 1980s; the cycle of post-war hospital construction which had caused a renewed cycle of modernization during the 1960s and 1970s had now run its course; inflationary interest rates discouraged institutions from taking on any new capital expenditures during the latter half of the 1970s and early 1980s; and the rise in the threshold which determines the number of projects that are reviewable was raised (between 1976 and 1979 all projects estimated to cost more than $150,000 were reviewable; as of 1981 projects of more than $600,000 were reviewable; currently only projects estimated at more than $2 million are reviewable). Thus, since fewer proposals were reviewable, the total sum of money being reported was reduced. Additionally, the increased threshold may have permitted institutions to parcel out their expenditures (if they did not involve adding ten or more beds) in order to avoid CON review altogether. Which, if any, of these possibilities applies is difficult to determine. My assessment, therefore, remains impressionistic.

There is evidence that the number of proposals coming to the Urban HSA declined over time. The rising threshold provides one obvious explanation; the cyclical nature of construction and the idea of pent-up demand provide other possibilities. It is also possible that a large share of the explanation for the decline in proposals can be attributed to the shift from in-patient care to ambulatory care being encouraged by pressure from third-party payers. (Such projects are not covered by CON in this state.) There were also rumors according to the staff, which no one was eager to verify, that a few hospitals were simply going ahead with construction without submitting proposals to the HSA.

The fact that such a large number of possibilities exists to explain why capital expenditures did not rise more than they did might be best interpreted to mean that health planning had a positive effect on cost containment over the past few years even if we don't know precisely which factor is responsible. However, these effects may not have come as a direct consequence of any of the actions taken by the planning agencies. In fact, to the extent that one highly publicized incident served as a test case of the teeth the Urban HSA had at its disposal, it became embarrassingly clear that its teeth may not have been the primary cause of its success in holding down expenditures. The test was staged when the executive director of the Urban HSA decided to challenge a large medical center hospital which increased its level of expenditure when it altered its plans during construction. The hospital had been involved in building an addition for about three years. As the new building came closer to completion, it became obvious that it was very expensive looking. The contrast between it and the area in which it was situated made its appearance even more striking. This flew in the face of public sentiments regarding health care costs according to newspaper reports which, in turn, provided the opportunity to raise questions about the HSA's effectiveness. The HSA director decided to confront the situation by calling a press conference to announce that the hospital had violated its CON agreement by: (1) permitting extensive cost overruns, (2) building an expensive ramp which was not approved, and (3) altering the original plans it submitted for approval by taking space away from an employee locker room and using this space to extend a laboratory facility which would now house expensive new equipment and personnel. All of this, the director pointed out, would be paid for out of increased patient charges. The Urban HSA's CON review committee was put in the position of having to call a special session to consider the situation. Media representatives were there to record the fact that the HSA was taking steps to control what the director was calling a flagrant violation of a contract with an agency charged with the responsibility of protecting the public's interests. Hospital representatives, who were also given the opportunity to comment publicly, responded by saying that the cost overruns were to be expected during an inflationary period; that the ramp was essential for transporting patients and really did not cost very much considering the advantages; and that advances in medical knowledge regarding the procedures to be performed in the new lab space could not have been predicted several years ago when the plans were being drawn up. Finally, the institution's spokesmen stated that as far as they were concerned they had followed procedures. There was no requirement that they report changes in their plans along the way to the HSA. (In fact, the federal law [PL 96–79] does require such a report, but the state statute does not clearly address this point; also, there was no precedent for this kind of event in the HSA's experience.)

The meeting called by the CON review committee to consider this problem was not a complete success because enough committee members did not show up to produce a quorum. The committee ended up recommending that the executive board censure the hospital involved. The board also did not have a quorum when it met a few days later because a number of people who did attend cited a conflict of interest and, therefore, could not vote on the motion to censure the hospital. The board sent a strongly worded recommendation to the state agency indicating the lack of a supporting vote for censure. The state agency meeting was exceptionally well attended that month. Both the hospital and the Urban HSA presented their respective cases. As a result, the state agency committee members determined that some sort of sanction was in order. The state agency required the hospital to set aside a certain sum of money for free patient care during the following year; but since the hospital had such an excellent reputation, it was decided that asking it to provide evidence that it had fulfilled this obligation was both unnecessary and offensive. Thus, the issue was closed.

From the point of view of the Urban HSA's staff, the agency had been publicly humiliated. The state agency's action indicated that the Urban HSA's teeth were very dull indeed. To what extent the representatives of other institutions who witnessed this event altered their view of the HSA's power is not clear. However, the fact that the agency's staff and the participants were demoralized was difficult to escape over the next two to three months.

Prior to this case, when the HSA's powers had not yet been tested, it was not entirely clear what would happen if the HSA chose to use the teeth it had at its disposal. The fact that this incident occurred in 1983 must also be noted. The timing of this test undoubtedly was a consideration in the state's decision not to apply more severe sanctions. After all, the health planning apparatus was not expected to survive much longer given the steps being taken by the Reagan administration.

2. Using access as a criterion to measure the Urban HSA's success is even more difficult for a number of reasons. For one, access data on a local basis are not available; if such data were available, it is not clear how they could be adjusted to account for use of services outside of the local area. Also, it takes time for people to change their health care-seeking behavior; when they do alter their behavior, it is not always clear to what the shift should be attributed. Finally, one of the most important considerations in evaluating access is the availability of funding for health care, a factor not within the scope of the HSA's influence. One added observation related to this point is worth mentioning. Even though increased access is one of the three main objectives identified by the prevailing health planning legislation, mention of the relationship between access and health planning is entirely absent from the health planning literature.

Increasing the health care resources available, that is, access, to the under-served was, nevertheless, one of the main aims of the participants in the Urban HSA. How successful were they in attaining this objective? Again, this is a matter of perspective. Some HSA participants were happier than others with what the HSA had achieved. No one was completely satisfied. There was, however, a high level of consensus, among participants as well as staff, about the reason why more was not achieved. First among the reasons was the fact that the HSA had to wait for proposals to come in; it could only react to proposals rather than having the power to stimulate or initiate proposals in areas that were underserved. There was also the widespread belief that the major institutions in the area would get their way in any case. The smaller institutions, which were providing only partial services and struggling to do so, posed a particularly difficult dilemma. Even though the guidelines would support denial of a proposal to expand a facility under such conditions, these were often the primary sources of care in underserved communities. In short, the HSA's performance using this criterion was only fair, largely because it was not equipped to address this objective very well.

3. Did the Urban HSA have an effect on the quality of care available? The original version of the law would have permitted the HSA to evaluate the "appropriateness" of the health care services in the area. However, the Health Planning and Development Act in its final form did not include such a provision. Instead, the HSA was mandated to consider quality in reviewing only those CON proposals that were presented to it outlining plans for expansion of services or facilities. Moreover, only the quality of services being addressed by the CON proposal were to be considered. Finally, the guidelines that specified the measures

to be used to evaluate a service were rather restrictive. The basic criterion required the institution to show that it had attained the recommended minimum number of procedures performed by the department under consideration and/or achieved the minimum occupancy level required. The only other means to affect quality that the agency had at its disposal was to deny an institution permission to institute certain clearly specified new services. The criteria for denying approval of a request to initiate a new service were based on the number of procedures performed together with the occupancy rates of other institutions in the area providing the service under consideration currently. Services not covered by the guidelines, which do not require new beds or expensive equipment, are not reviewable, and more direct measures of quality were not included in the legislation. (For a review of suggested indicators, see Hershey and Robinson 1981.)

There were few proposals to begin an entirely new service submitted during the time I spent at the HSA. No doubt this was due to the same reasons that dampened enthusiasm for submitting proposals outlining any form of expansion. In essence, the social climate of the times was not conducive to expansion. There was only one case in which quality considerations played a notable part. It involved a proposal to open a new open heart surgery unit.

Discussion on this proposal began when the newly appointed cardiac surgeon from a relatively small community hospital requested an appointment with the HSA staff to discuss the proposal on an informal basis. The hospital involved had developed an unsavory reputation based on a highly publicized refusal to accept an accident victim brought to its emergency room who died en route to another hospital in one instance, and, in another instance, a badly botched case of minor cosmetic surgery case which left the patient completely paralyzed and barely able to speak. (The patient was featured on the evening news many times approximately a year prior to this time.) Although the hospital had been taken over by another organization, changed its name, and had installed an entirely new staff, the unsavory reputation lingered. The cardiac surgeon, who arrived for the meeting accompanied by two senior hospital administrators, began by stating that the hospital was now a first-rate institution with ties to an important university medical center across town. He added that the university hospital would not have dealings with a small community hospital unless it met the high standards of the university hospital. He then described what the new unit he envisioned would be able to accomplish. He did not lack confidence in his own abilities, nor was he reluctant to describe his extensive talents in detail. The HSA staff members listened but were definitely not encouraging. They pointed out that other hospitals were closing down services which performed diagnostic workups preparatory to heart surgery, so it was unlikely that a new service could be sustained. The surgeon was not to be discouraged and argued that the area in which his hospital was located included many elderly patients who would benefit from heart surgery. When a staff person stated that several major institutions, which performed heart surgery regularly, were readily accessible, the surgeon countered by arguing that he could perform the same kind of surgery at a lower cost. The high cost of surgery, he said, was preventing many patients from availing themselves of this highly beneficial form of treatment. This, he stated triumphantly, would be a deficiency he would overcome. The meeting ended with the HSA staff people stating that the guidelines would not permit them to recommend a new open heart service unless institutions currently performing heart surgery increased their volume to such an extent that they could not cope. There was no reason to think this would happen in the near future. The surgeon was visibly irritated by the lack of enthusiasm being exhibited by the HSA staff. He said he would persist in spite of this response.

After he left, the staff members' assessment of the surgeon and his plans can be summed up in the following statement: "That guy is crazy!" Apart from discussion about the obvious lack of need for the service the surgeon was proposing based on the guidelines, there was also discussion regarding the quality that would result if a heart surgery unit were to open in a small institution, across town from the major medical center which was to provide backup in special cases.

When the completed proposal arrived, the staff gave it a negative appraisal, based strictly on criteria related to the need for such a service. There might have been room for a more positive review had quality not been a consideration. However, the decision had to be made based on the evidence at hand. It was made in the abstract rather than in reaction to concrete evidence on quality, which could only be obtained after the fact, that is, an established performance record in this particular institution. Would the unit have proved beneficial if it had been permitted to open? Were there people who would have benefited? Or would the new service have added to the cost of care by bringing in patients whose need for surgery was questionable or performed at some risk? Such questions will never be answered in this case.

Cases such as this one are, however, responsible for some of the negative characterizations of health planning that exist. For example, this case can also be used to illustrate the common criticism that health planning encourages "franchising." This means that competition from newcomers is discouraged by the HSA, which tends to protect the established institutions and, at the same time, reduce the incentive to develop more innovative approaches to care.

The final hearing on the proposal for a new heart surgery service also deserves some comment. When the time came for the surgeon to make his remarks, he gave full vent to his frustration. He accused the HSA staff of being rude, insulting, and totally set against the proposal from the outset. It is true that the staff members made some unkind remarks about this man but they did not do so to his face. However, he had no one else at whom to lash out. He was angry because the HSA staff was unimpressed with his personal ambitions. He chose to launch a vituperative attack on the staff members; however, he chose the wrong approach. The HSA participants took offense at the surgeon's remarks because the negative comments reflected on the performance of the agency as a whole. The case left everyone involved with a bad taste. The surgeon undoubtedly will tell his colleagues about his experience, citing it as evidence that health planning is a disaster; while the HSA consumer representatives, staff, as well as a few of the provider representatives will remember this as an illustration of provider domination they successfully resisted.

CONCLUSIONS REGARDING THE URBAN HSA: PERFORMANCE

In the final analysis, to the extent that the Urban HSA was successful on any dimension, what factors can be said to be responsible for its success? In my judgment, the handful of respondents who said that "things would have been worse without the HSA" came closest to the answer. As far as cost containment is concerned, the fact that the HSA was simply "there" and charged with conducting CON reviews in and of itself produced certain changes. One of the changes was the care which went into preparing plans involving capital expenditures. Initially, hospitals could not be sure how stringent this new set of controls would be. What was certain, however, was that an institution's plans were now open to the public, meaning at minimum that anyone interested in examining them could do so. In order to avoid negative publicity when the topic of cost control seemed to be attracting a considerable amount of public attention, hospitals had to take care in thinking through and presenting their plans. In short, many factors, some more tangible than others, played a part in the cost containment performance of the Urban HSA. However, the major share of the credit must, in my judgment, be attributed to something as intangible as the social context of the time, which the HSA embodied, rather than crediting any of the specific actions that it may have taken. The fact of the matter is that the power of the HSA was more impressive when it was still in the form of an unspecified threat than it was once it moved from the level of threat to the level of action.

In my estimation, the Urban HSA appeared to be more successful when there was a high level of general social support for controlling the health care system via a health planning approach. When support was withdrawn, as evidenced by talk of dismantling the program and reductions in funding, the approach lost credibility, and the HSA's power declined proportionately. To the extent that it succeeded in meeting the objectives that it sought to achieve, its success was due to the strength of the belief that the HSA had a good deal of power, which would be backed up by some unspecified long arm of government in Washington. Its successes were less directly related to any particular manifestation of its powers.

It is also true that power in this form posed a greater threat to some institutions than to others. The large, university-affiliated institutions operate in circles which make the threat of government sanctions less ominous. Numerous individuals in such institutions in the HSA planning area have ties to Washington through various funding agencies, important political figures, as well as networks of influentials in other institutions. The result is an image of Washington's power in human proportions. The image of power conjured up by smaller institutions is less palpable and, therefore, more threatening. The smaller institutions, having few alternatives, appealed for mercy and understanding at the hands of the HSA.

Evidence to support this observation comes from reminiscences about the "good old days." When the history of the Urban HSA was recounted by the staff and some of the participants of long-standing, it became clear that the composition of the HSA committees had changed over time. In the first few years of its existence, the HSA was able to enroll high status provider representatives from the major institutions in the area. Over time they stopped attending. To the extent such institutions were represented when I arrived, more often than not the representatives were recruited from the middle layers of these organizations. My interpretation of this drop in interest among high status providers is that the initial wave of concern about the ability of the administrative system of control to affect the plans being made by major institutions had subsided along with the wave of anticipatory capital investment, which had also run its course. In short, several trends were coinciding—funds for capital expansion had become too costly; much capital expansion had been completed earlier when the need for such expenditures was more acute (Medicare and Medicaid required institutions to use two-person rooms instead of wards; thus, beds, monitoring equipment, as well as roofs, and such, were updated during this major remodeling phase); and the representatives of major institutions were anticipating the shift in social climate away from a regulatory system of control, which was receiving a steady stream of early negative evaluation, in favor of the market system of control.

Additionally, the major institutions took steps to ensure against problems in future dealings with the HSA by hiring away HSA staff members. All of the staff members who left the Urban HSA accepted positions with large hospitals or with consulting firms; a former chairman of the executive board accepted a position with a hospital management consulting firm whose services were used on a number of occasions in preparing proposals. The director of the agency left by the end of my study to start his own consulting firm. In effect, the Urban HSA, as did other HSAs, trained both the regulators and their counterparts who were employed by the institutions that were being regulated. In fact, a large association of health planners now exists to bring together planners from both sides to discuss their work and the means they will use to protect their shared interest in sustaining health planning as a viable occupation.

Part III

Summary and Implications

9

Conclusions

After reviewing the record of health planning in the United States over the twentieth century, what I find most striking is the high level of consensus present among the majority of those concerned (consumers, providers, vendors, evaluators, and such) regarding the need for major changes in current health care delivery arrangements. Equally striking is the complete lack of consensus past this point when it comes to identifying the problem and its solution. This situation is clearly illustrated by public survey data showing that a majority of the public considers the health care system to be in a state of crisis and that there is little consensus regarding the aspects that should be changed. In my estimation, the persistent perception of a health crisis stems from society's lack of confidence in the social control arrangements governing the activities of the health sector in recent years; what is worse is that the public is confused about who should be entrusted with the responsibility for planning the nation's health (Mead 1977). The primary reason for the confusion is the paucity of information to assist in altering the current situation (Ermann 1976). This is not to say that the relevant information does not exist; however, the existing information is poorly organized, inaccessible, and uneven. In actuality a great deal of information is being generated, but it is often disseminated in a way that adds to the public's sense of confusion (Evans 1983).

This chapter consolidates a portion of the vast amount of information available in the hope of reducing some of the confusion surrounding current discourse regarding the problems affecting the health sector. (For another perspective see the APHA Presidential Address, Addiss 1985.) The discussion presented here begins with a review of the topics addressed in preceding chapters. Outlined is the sequence of steps responsible for the design of the health care delivery system that now exists. Then the evidence available on the performance of the mechanisms associated with each of the social control arrangements experienced to date is discussed. Next, the special features of the health sector and the effects that these characteristics have had on continuing efforts to plan for the nation's health are considered. This portion of the discussion serves as the background against which to examine the strengths and weaknesses of the three available systems of social control. Finally, my own opinion regarding the best approach to social control is offered.

THE OVERVIEW OF PLANNING FOR THE NATION'S HEALTH

Based on the historical overview presented in earlier chapters, we can see that the central focus of health planning shifted several times. During the early part of the twentieth century, health planning efforts were primarily directed toward improving the quality of health care. This goal remained intact until the nation experienced nearly a decade of post–World War II reconstruction, at which point society began turning its attention to internal social problems, especially the existence of social inequity. Accordingly, the health planning goal was altered to encompass equal access to health care services. The pursuit of high quality in the delivery of health care remained an integral part of the goal. By the 1970s the goal was again redefined to include the aim of delivering health care at a reasonable cost. Within a few years this portion of the goal was revised to focus on a more ambitious objective—cost containment. By 1980, the goal was altered for the fourth time during the twentieth century. Now the new component was not given a commonly agreed-upon label. However, it is clear that what is being demanded at present is improved efficiency, specifically, managerial efficiency. Thus, the goal currently serving to guide the activities of the health sector includes the following components: (1) the highest quality of care possible, (2) access to health services for everyone, and (3) cost containment, (4) which is to be achieved by encouraging or, if necessary, forcing the health sector to incorporate the principles of managerial efficiency.

The timing involved in these shifts is significant. Note that the initial goal, quality, set forth early in this century was not altered for approximately five decades and that the three new components were added between the mid 1960s and the early 1980s. The fact that the goal of quality remained unaltered for so long indicates that society was reasonably satisfied with this health care objective and with the leadership provided by the medical profession in attaining it. The logical corollary of this observation is that the subsequent alterations indicate persistent social dissatisfaction with the performance of the health sector.

We must look to the "social climate" prevailing during particular periods of time to find the best single explanation for shifts in satisfaction with the health care system over the course of the twentieth century. To illustrate, during the era when the pursuit of quality gave the health sector its primary purpose, a number of other matters emerged to capture society's attention, namely, two world wars and a major economic depression, overshadowing for periods of time society's concern about health care. At the same time, the course that medical progress was taking matched prevailing social values holding scientific/techno-logical progress and expertise in high regard. Accordingly, the medical profession received the credit for the progress that was being achieved by the health sector. The shift in social values that occurred during the early 1960s came in response to the recognition that the sense of well-being and prosperity that followed World War II did not extend to all Americans. Society responded by launching into action on a variety of fronts (in addition to an expanding military front in Vietnam). Such newly recognized social problems as poverty, social inequality, the plight of the elderly, and the financial devastation caused by prolonged illness provided the agenda for social action. The reluctance of the medical profession to embrace the solutions being developed at this time was responsible, at least in part, for planting the seeds of social dissatisfaction with the prevailing health sector arrangements that had been governed without interference by the medical profession for so long.

Two added factors, to which the emergence of social dissatisfaction can be attributed, are rooted in the increase in funding plus the rise in expectations about personal health status that accompanied the newly identified social priorities of the 1960s. The massive influx of federal funds produced well-known effects— the overall expenditures on health care increased, health care facilities and ser-vices multiplied, the pool of health care workers expanded at an unprecedented rate, the technology employed by the health sector became more sophisticated and expensive, and so on. In combination, the ready availability of government monies plus a strong sense of social support for the development of the health care sector attracted a high level of investment in terms of personal energy and private funds. (To illustrate, expansion occurred among the following: medical schools, medical specialty societies, across the allied health occupations, health administrators, quasi-government agencies, third-party payers, equipment man-ufacturers, hospital supply companies, contractors of services to health care institutions, plus the vast array of special-interest consumer groups.) It is im-portant to recognize, however, that those who developed a vested interest in this sector did so in response to prevailing social values and incentives. That this high level of involvement would pose a problem in time was not anticipated. Nevertheless, the fact that so many diverse groups developed vested interests in the health sector indicates that these groups also have reason to protect their respective interests and investments.

Even so, the large number of parties involved would be less problematic if not for the apparent inability of the health sector to make much headway in addressing the problem of rising costs. The situation has now come full circle. Commonly agreed-upon problems have become increasingly more difficult to resolve because so many different interest groups have become involved, each holding vastly different ideas regarding the solutions to address those problems. Even those who agree on a general approach to a problem differ on the specifics when their respective vested interests are threatened. Clearly, the large number and the diversity of interested parties is now exacerbating the situation.

Thus, while the shifts in health care goals over the past few decades are related to the increasing complexity of this sector, it is the continuous rise in health costs that is primarily responsible for the idea that the health sector is growing in an uncontrolled and poorly managed fashion. This assessment coexists with the recognition that the rate at which medical knowledge is being advanced is awesome. Not commonly acknowledged, but possibly of greater significance to the effort to achieve greater control over the health sector, is the fact that no one devoting time and energy to the pursuit of medical knowledge or its application is willing to abandon this work without a fight. Nor are any of the other members of organizations whose livelihood depends upon the continuity of health sector pursuits prepared to step aside. The consumers of health care services are certainly not ready to accept any reductions when their own health care is involved. Yet, we as a society are now being pressed to confront choices which will inevitably affect negatively some category of participants if health care costs are to be curbed to any extent.

The enthusiasm with which institutions in the health care sector have taken steps ostensibly intended to increase efficiency would seem to indicate that a consensus has been reached regarding the preferred means to use in addressing the complex health care goal as it is currently defined. However, I anticipate that the most recent approach introduced, the market system of control, will provide only a relatively temporary solution, at least in its current form. The sudden interest in this approach coincides with the shift in social values signaled by the election of Ronald Reagan. We are now in a period during which the pursuit of self-interest is being advocated as the best means to attain collective goals (Thurow 1985). Reducing the role assigned to government in favor of an increased role for the private sector, a trend currently known as "privatization," is a central feature of this approach. The reason this approach may not turn out to be a long-lived solution is that a steadily growing faction of persons who favored this approach are shifting their loyalties as their own jobs are eliminated in the competitive marketplace (for example, farmers, steelworkers, auto workers, bankers). Commentators speaking about problems associated with the national economy point to the Reagan administration's inability to deal with the national deficit and its impact on an entire range of social priorities. The fact that this approach has not been as successful as its advocates promised it would be is certain to rekindle unresolved debates about the value of regulatory versus market controls in some sectors, the health sector in particular (Vladek 1985). This assessment should not be interpreted to mean, however, that I am advocating that any of the newly introduced mechanisms aimed at curbing health care costs should be abandoned. After all, one of the major lessons learned from the experience of health planning is that the performance of control mechanisms improves over time and with experience. We learned this as we learned to carry out the evaluation procedures themselves. It is to the literature that I now turn.

EVALUATIONS OF HEALTH PLANNING PERFORMANCE

While an historical overview allows us to consider health planning over the entire twentieth century, the literature evaluating its performance is largely a product of the past three decades. In effect, health planning, as practiced over the first half of this century, the era during which the medical profession was basically responsible for planning society's health care, has not been scrutinized in the same way that it has been over the last thirty years, nor have we had enough time and experience with the market approach to health planning to have accrued comparable data on its performance. In fact, what we have is a considerable amount of information on the successes and failures of one approach to social control, the administrative approach. As a result, any effort to draw comparisons across the three systems of control, which is of central interest to the discussion presented in this book, must be treated with caution. With this caveat in mind, let us examine the data available.

The health planning literature of the past thirty years provides two sets of answers to the question: What have we learned from our experience with health planning? One branch of this literature is concerned with health planning outcomes, measured in terms of cost savings. The other branch focuses on the planning process but is primarily interested in the issue of participation. From the perspective of those who are primarily interested in planning outcomes, health planning attained little success in containing costs during the early years of administrative planning (the mid 1960s through the mid 1970s). However, there is evidence to indicate that substantial savings were being attained just at the time when administrative control was about to be superseded by the market system of control (the late 1970s and early 1980s). The researchers who focus on planning outcomes offer two main reasons for this. First, gains in experience attained by planning agencies over time resulted in increased effectiveness; second, it was determined that earlier findings indicating poor results in containing costs were based on premature and faulty data. The second answer regarding what we have learned comes from the portion of the health planning literature focusing on the process of planning. This portion of the literature states that the problems surrounding participation in the planning process were never satisfactorily resolved.

The case study findings presented here offer a third perspective. I am not suggesting that the findings revealed by a single case study can be treated as if they apply to all or, for that matter, any other health planning agency. The case study does proceed, however, from a foundation laid by the existing literature; and, to that extent, the conclusions found in the existing literature serve as a framework for considering the case study findings. The primary contribution that the discussion based on the case study makes is to introduce a previously neglected dimension, the structural dimension, into discussions aimed at evaluating the success of health planning efforts.

To the extent that the case study attempted to address questions stimulated by the existing literature, the conclusions found in the literature on the process of health planning were found to be only partly applicable. Because one of the earliest hurdles that the health planning effort encountered revolved around determining who should participate in the planning process, this became an early legislative concern as well. Health planning participants were viewed as members of two separate categories—providers or consumers. Legislative measures were aimed at increasing the influence of consumers, an aim consistent with the prevailing belief that one of the primary problems confronting health planning at that time was provider domination. The division of participants into two categories was built on the assumption that consumers and providers would see themselves as members of two distinct groups, who would also embrace the respective identities assigned to them and behave accordingly in the health planning forum. In effect, the portion of the health planning legislation that dealt with participation was based on a two-party decision making model. In the case of the Urban HSA, the expectations inherent in this model were not fulfilled.

While coalitions based on shared political interests did emerge among the Urban HSA participants, they did not fit the two-party model, at least not in the way the designers of the legislation which created HSAs had anticipated. Consumers and providers united to form coalitions around community boundaries. In the Urban HSA area, community interest was synonymous with racial/ethnic community interest, which, in turn, generally approximated geographic community boundaries. A number of coalitions of this kind evolved to overshadow the anticipated consumer-provider split.

This is not to say that the differences between the interests and agendas that the consumers and providers, respectively, brought to bear on the Urban HSA planning process were irrelevant. There were readily identifiable differences in the way that members of these two categories saw the basic problems that were presented before them as well as the expectations they had regarding what they hoped to accomplish. Generally, these differences closely reflected an individual's familiarity with the workings of the health care delivery system. The more experience an individual had, the more comprehensive were the changes that the individual thought were necessary. The less familiarity an individual brought to the process, the less extensive were the changes envisioned. This explains why the consumers, who were generally less knowledgeable about the workings of the health care system, could express a higher level of satisfaction about the Urban HSA's achievements.

The case study was not specifically designed to confirm or reject the findings presented by the literature, particularly the outcome-oriented literature, much of which is concerned with the problems inherent in measuring cost savings. However, the general discussion found in this portion of the literature includes rich, descriptive analyses of the difficulties agencies encountered in attempting to achieve savings, in which so many varied problems are mentioned that at least some of them apply to the Urban HSA situation. Furthermore, the most generally agreed-upon conclusion found in this literature fits the Urban HSA case very well, namely, that greater cost savings were attained as the participants and staff gained experience. The major reservations expressed in this literature regarding the difficulty of analyzing data to support such a conclusion apply in this case equally well. Much of the difficulty stems from the fact that the conditions under which the health planning agencies were operating were themselves undergoing change over the period of time under consideration. For example, the law governing health planning was revised; an economic recession made capital funding more difficult to obtain, which had an impact on the capital expenditures hospitals were willing to undertake; a shift toward ambulatory care was just beginning to gain momentum with its own effects on costs and so on.

One of the most important observations to be made about the health planning literature is that it grew out of two separate disciplinary bases—economics and political science—and that the two disciplines have had no particular need to speak to each other on this topic. While their respective conclusions have been moving toward a common ground, there has been little effort to integrate them. The attempt to do so yields an interesting, logical by-product which deserves some consideration. Consider, first, the fact that the outcome of health planning, measured in terms of cost savings, was, in the final analysis, judged to be a positive one, the consensus being that increased experience contributed substantially to bringing about this outcome. If, however, the major conclusion of the other branch of the literature is that participation in the process of planning was never satisfactorily resolved, whose growth in experience should be credited for the successful outcomes that eventually resulted? It seems we are left with only one conclusion—it was the HSA staff that benefited by the gains in experience. The Urban HSA case study data lend some support to this interpretation.

The Urban HSA participants used the term "streamlining" to explain how the staff in recent years had begun to manage the enormous amount of paper that participants were expected to read. Over time the staff reduced the amount of paper being sent to participants by reducing the number of original documents and expanding the staff summary portions of the mailing. As the staff members became more experienced in interpreting the law and codifying the abstract goals, the agency became more efficient.

It is difficult to know, of course, where the natural course of this trend toward increased efficiency would have led had funding and social support for the administrative approach been continued. The classic sociological literature on organizations leads us to expect increasing formalization, organizational entrenchment, greater adherence to rules, and more reliance on an impersonal approach to complicated issues, that is, a bureaucratic operating format. As it is, the Urban HSA's future is in doubt because its funding has been steadily declining and its mandate whittled away. Under these conditions it is not surprising to find that interest in its own survival is moving to the forefront of the Urban HSA's list of concerns.

The more closely one scrutinizes the workings of this or any other health planning agency, the larger the number of organizational problems associated with the administrative approach to control one is likely to find. However, different but equally problematic organizational problems should be expected to appear if either of the other two available systems of control were to replace the administrative control system.

It is interesting, therefore, that current debates about the superiority of one mechanism of control versus another are often based on empirical data documenting the flaws of the administrative approach, while the salutary effects that can be expected from as yet untested mechanisms associated with the market approach are grounded in promises. Even more interesting is the fact that such debates generally proceed without objections raised by anyone regarding the unevenness of the bases on which the argument is constructed.

In short, each approach for imposing greater control available to us brings with it its own strengths and weaknesses. Before discussing these, however, I would like to point out that any approach to control we select must operate within the context provided by the special features of the health care delivery system. It is to the relationship between these characteristics and health planning efforts that I now turn.

HEALTH SECTOR CHARACTERISTICS

It seems that everyone who comments on the workings of the health sector points to one or another aspect which makes it difficult to achieve greater order or control over this sector. There also are those whose primary purpose is to describe the characteristics of the health care system. Few go on to draw connections between the two. Consider the relationship between the characteristics of the health care sector and the effort to bring order to it. Although the exercise of describing these features could easily serve as the main topic of a lengthy volume, my purpose is more circumscribed. I direct my attention to a limited number of characteristics, those I believe pose the greatest constraints: (1) the size of the health sector, (2) its institutional structure, (3) the nature of the goal involved, (4) the factor of continuous change, and (5) its financial potential.

Size

That the health sector expanded rapidly and is now very large are facts that are mentioned often in passing. The indicator that is most commonly used in referring to the size of the health sector is the percentage of the GNP (Gross National Product) that is devoted to health. This figure troubles most those who are fully cognizant of the meaning of the GNP (the measure of all goods and services exchanged in the society). The public seems to view the rising level of the GNP devoted to health as far too distant from its personal purse to cause concern (Altman and Blendon 1984). In recent years, however, another portion of the GNP for which the government bears sole responsibility, defense, has also been growing. The fact that the proportion devoted to both is increasing is

Table 5
Fiscal Trends in the National Budget

Year	National Health Expenditures	National Defense Expenditures
1950[1]	4.4	4.7
1960[2]	5.3	9.7
1965	6.1	7.7
1970	7.6	8.4
1975	8.6	5.8
1980	9.4	5.2
1981	9.7	5.5
1982	10.5	6.1
1983	10.8	6.5
1984	10.6[3]	6.7

[1]U.S. Bureau of the Census, Statistical Abstract of the United States, 1985, 105th ed. (Washington, D.C., 1984), pp. 96, 331.

[2]Ibid., 1984, 104th ed. (Washington, D.C., 1983), pp. 102, 343.

[3]Health United States, 1985, U.S. Department of Health and Human Services (Washington, D.C., 1986), p. 128.

a source of great concern to those who have reason to be interested in the national budget. Consider the trends exhibited in Table 5.

The significance of the continued expansion in the size of the health sector requires little interpretation. The larger and more dispersed an enterprise is, the more difficult it is to coordinate and direct the efforts of that enterprise in a systematic manner. Understanding the relationship among the structures through which it operates is essential if greater order and control are to be achieved (Ermann 1976).

Institutional Structure

One especially important feature of the health care sector is one which is also not readily apparent, namely, the absence of centralized institutional structures that might represent the interest groups involved. This is not to suggest that such structures would not have serious drawbacks were they to come into existence. However, the lack of centralized structures makes discussion among the parties involved disorganized and inefficient. There are, of course, a number of organizations that play central roles within the health sector. The AMA quickly comes to mind as the organization which speaks for the medical profession. However, as I have pointed out previously, if only 30% of practicing physicians are enrolled, can it truly be said that the AMA represents the whole medical profession? The American Hospital Association (AHA), by contrast, does represent the vast majority of hospitals. However, the constituency it represents is highly heterogeneous, including small rural hospitals, major medical center hospitals, privately owned chains of hospitals, and so forth. Thus, like the AMA, it must maintain a stance which is not highly specific in order to satisfy its wide-ranging membership. There is also the organization representing for-profit hospitals, the Federation of American Hospitals. Not surprisingly, its aims do not always coincide with the aims of other groups within this sector. The public, for its part, has no single representative, and the special interest consumer groups who do have organized representation generally do not attempt to co-ordinate their efforts. Nor can the companies whose profit margins are closely connected to developments taking place in this sector turn to a single repre-sentative organization. In short, a multitude of unrelated organizations can be identified representing the interests of virtually everyone with a stake in this sector, but there is little interaction among them. In the meantime, the individual redress of perceived injustices is pursued via the courts with increasing frequency and with steadily escalating awards.

Clearly the disadvantage in this arrangement is that a consensus regarding changes in the policy and practices governing the delivery of health care services is difficult to achieve. This is true not only because differences in opinion are inevitable, but there is no single place to hold a discussion to address those differences. Nor does a recognized set of representatives exist that is limited to manageable numbers and legitimated through any of the traditional means, such as election to office in a representational organization. On the other hand, the fact that little effort has been made to alter these arrangements suggests that the advantages of this inefficient arrangement outweigh the disadvantages for many, if not all, concerned. The advantages include the freedom to address problems at the level where they occur, generally at the juncture where the providers of health services and the consumers of those services interact. A radical alteration in these arrangements is unlikely unless several categories of participants de-termine that there are advantages in unification. If, however, one coalition were to emerge that threatened to unbalance the current situation in which the power to affect changes in the structure of the health care delivery system is broadly diffused, then other coalitions could be expected to develop in rapid succession.

There are some signs that the coalition formation process may have begun. When it was recognized that the attempt to tighten the federal budget was causing the burden of costs to be shifted to the private sector, the private insurance industry responded with tighter controls of its own. Furthermore, it is generally expected that the DRG reimbursement schedule, which currently covers Medicare patients only, will be extended to cover all categories of patients. In fact, DRG scales of payment are already being phased-in to cover Medicaid admissions in a number of states. As third party reimbursement evolves toward increased uniformity, few avenues except unified resistance will be left to those providers of health services who feel that some part of the reimbursement schedule is too restrictive or inappropriate on other grounds. Thus far, physicians have responded individualistically by reducing their participation or joining groups willing to assume the responsibility for negotiating payment with third-party payers. How-ever, judging from the experiences of other countries which have imposed stricter controls over reimbursements (for example, the Canadian provinces, especially

Ontario and Quebec, as well as the United Kingdom), we should not be surprised if the medical profession takes steps to unify its forces in order to negotiate from a position of strength (Woods 1986).

The attempts of hospital administrators to arrive at a unified response to government efforts to tighten controls have been complicated by the fact that some hospitals are sustaining significant financial losses while others are prospering. This is not to say that hospital administrators have been passive (Zuckerman 1983). The past five years have witnessed the emergence of hospital chains on both the not-for-profit as well as the for-profit sides of the industry; urgent care and ambulatory care centers have sprung up everywhere; vigorous marketing has suddenly become commonplace, and so on. The internal organization of hospitals also has been undergoing some change. Although conflicts between administrators and physicians remain, an increasing number of hospital boards of directors and executive boards have been inviting physicians into their inner circles. It would seem that if efforts to contain health care costs continue to be as vigorously implemented in the future as they have in the past year or two, some hospital administrators and doctors will be readier to acknowledge that they have a shared interest in combining their efforts to ensure the viability of their hospital's future (Shortell, Morrisey, and Conrad 1985).

It is interesting to consider the irony in this situation. When health planning was organized around an administrative approach to control, one of the built-in assumptions was that the providers would act in response to a sense of "consciousness of kind." This assumption did not materialize. Now that the health sector has moved toward a market system of control, the prevailing assumption is that providers will be motivated to compete with one another rather than to join forces. However, if providers perceive themselves to be competing for a limited number of dollars and constricted by a fixed schedule of reimbursements, then it should not be too surprising if they develop a characteristic usually associated with groups: a recognition of the existence of shared interests which stand in opposition to the interests of those who control third party payments, thereby creating clear boundaries dividing "them" from those who will now see themselves as "us."

THE NATURE OF THE GOAL

The third characteristic of the health sector with which any system of control must contend is the nature of the goal involved. Consider what we as a society want to set forth as the ultimate goal toward which we expect the health care delivery system to work. To date we have identified a four-part goal: improving the quality of health care, ensuring that all persons in the society have access to health care, containing the ever-increasing costs of care, and making certain that health care is being delivered in the most efficient manner possible. It is worth noting that improving the health of society is not one of the goals we have set forth for ourselves. Of course, it has always been the ultimate goal we hoped to achieve. Improving the health of society is, however, far too abstract an objective to function as a stated goal. It is too difficult to measure, especially in the short run; one can never be sure that one's current efforts will bring about the desired results in the future; at the very least, one cannot guarantee the best avenue for arriving at the final goal is being followed. For these reasons intermediate goals have been identified. In practice, however, the four intermediate goals now guiding the efforts of the health care sector suffer from some of the same problems from which the ultimate goal of improving the nation's health suffers.

Much of the current confusion about goal attainment revolves around the measures that the government should take in support of one step or another. The confusion stems from the fact that discussion is invariably introduced with the promise that the measure in question will improve the delivery of health care for all. Which step is, in fact, the best is unclear because all the measures recommended are of necessity based on theoretical assumptions and promises which can only be tested via implementation in the arena where people's health and attitudes about health care will be directly affected. For obvious reasons those in a position to influence action are wary of risking a miscalculation. At present, this is largely the province of our representatives in the federal government because the government pays the largest portion of the nation's health care bill. In order to achieve support for their respective agendas, each set of advocates is appealing to the public, urging the public to register directly or indirectly its support for that particular measure with its political representatives. Thus, we have a situation where a variety of interested parties is appealing to the public, each with its own agenda, criticisms, and alternative objectives. The result is apparent when the public is surveyed regarding its views on the health care delivery system. The consensus is that there is something seriously wrong with the system, but it is not at all clear exactly what the problem is or what should be done about it. Obviously, there would be far less confusion about the preferred solution to the problem if the problem was more clearly identifiable. The reason it is not is that so many different parties are offering competing interpretations. In short, the nature of the goal guiding the activities of the health sector exerts a powerful influence on the operations of this sector. If the goal were less abstract and ambiguous, it might be easier to arrive at a consensus regarding an operational measure to gauge our performance in moving toward that goal. As it is, the vigor with which competing interpretations are being promoted is likely to continue because of the size of the stakes involved, including such traditional rewards as money, individual as well as institutional autonomy, status and power.

CONTINUOUS CHANGE

The fact that the health care delivery system operates in an atmosphere of continuous change is a fourth factor making the effort to bring order to this sector difficult. Although planning under conditions of change is not an unusual operating constraint, the rate of change combined with the scope of health care sector endeavors mean that this characteristic deserves special attention. I will focus on three dimensions of change particularly troublesome now: (a) demographic trends, particularly the aging of the population, (b) the rate of expansion in technological capability, and (c) the impact of changes in social values.

(a) The effects that the aging of the population is having on the health care sector are well known. With increasing age, individuals are more likely to suffer chronic illness, increase their visits to physicians, spend more days receiving in-patient care, and so on. This increased use of services translates into increased costs. Since government programs (Medicare and Medicaid) provide coverage for anyone over sixty-five years of age, the steady expansion of this population has been reflected in a growing bill for health care. The sense of urgency about addressing this problem is being spurred on by two other factors in the list of changing conditions—the rapid expansion of medical technological capability and changing social values with regard to the elderly on the one hand, and medical technology on the other.

(b) Increasing technological capability means that health providers are able to select among a much larger range of techniques, especially life-sustaining techniques, and use them to benefit the portion of the population which is the fastest growing portion and exhibits the highest utilization rates.

At the same time, the ability to sustain life at the other end of the life cycle, in the case of seriously ill and impaired infants, is adding to the sudden and unprecedented increase in the number of critically ill persons who use the most expensive forms of health care services. While the benefits this increasing technological capability has brought along with it in terms of expanded medical knowledge are being greeted with awe and gratitude by medical researchers and members of society at large, the problems associated with the same advances are impossible to ignore. We have here a perfect example of "cultural lag." Our technological capability in this instance has far outpaced our ability to integrate that technology into the culture. We have not developed the norms necessary to govern the application of the new forms of highly sophisticated technology or the values that give meaning to the effects produced by the technology.

(c) The third arena of change that affects the functioning of the health care sector is formed by the point at which social values intersect with financial costs. As medical technological capability increases and the population affected continues to expand, questions regarding the cost versus the benefit of administering state-of-the-art treatment are intruding into discussions in a growing number of cases.

There are few commonly agreed upon guidelines to assist either the providers of care or the families of seriously ill persons in determining how extensive treatment should be. This is because we do not have a fully developed set of values and norms which would come into play under such circumstances. To illustrate, most people espouse the idea that death with dignity is a highly valued social good. Yet, if there is some doubt regarding the point at which death occurs, then it is also not clear when life sustaining equipment stops sustaining life and begins to prolong dying. We are not sure whether we should say to ourselves that employing heroic measures in cases where death is inevitable causes unnecessary suffering to the person and detracts from the peace that should come when a life is ending, or if we should say that hope should never be abandoned if there is even the slightest chance that death can be forestalled. The former position is sometimes supported by the argument that resources are being wasted because physicians wish to aggrandize their egos by assuming godlike control over life-and-death decisions. The argument states that medical resources could be better used to prevent illness than to intervene after it is clear that death is inevitable. The alternative stance lends itself to arguing that a cure could be discovered at the last minute and the course of the illness reversed just in time, and that all life-saving efforts should be made under virtually all circumstances because there is nothing more precious than a human life. Finally, since no one has the right to play God, no one has the right to withdraw technological support even if the person is only surviving with the assistance of machines.

Those who espouse the latter stance generally dismiss the issue of costs as inconsequential in contrast to the value of human life. This leaves those who oppose what they see as excessive technological intervention in a far more difficult position. In stating that the costs of employing heroic measures are too high and that there are better uses for those resources, this faction is put in the position of having to identify preferable ways of using those funds. The most commonly proposed alternative is that funds should be shifted away from acute care to benefit preventive care, not a particularly controversial idea. However, while many may agree in principle that there might be some value to this idea, a major shift in this portion of expenditures is not likely because there is so much vested interest in the segment of the health sector involved in delivering acute care. The discussion becomes more threatening when the statement is made that our health care resources are not unlimited. If scarcity is acknowledged, then the question of distribution moves to the forefront of the discussion. As long as we as a society refuse to admit that scarcity is an issue, we can avoid the need to confront sensitive discussions concerned with distribution. However, this topic is cropping up with increasing regularity. If there is a shortage of organs, who should be the first to receive one? Should heroic (that is, expensive) measures be used to save people whose life expectancy is very short in any case (that is, the aged)? This leads to the question of how old is too old to be saved using heroic measures? Should extraordinary efforts be made to save the severely damaged child of a poor, unwed, inadequately educated teenaged mother, whose ability to care for the child is doubtful once the child is released from the hospital? In short, are some people's lives worth more than others'? Should life-worth be entered into a cost-benefit equation? How else can we allocate scarce resources? Few models are available from which to choose.

According to Henry Aaron and William Schwartz (1984), the British resolve these questions by allowing physicians to allocate scarce resources at their own discretion. Their decisions are not questioned because everyone shares the basic values that govern decisions in this area, including the fact that after a certain age, say fifty-five, one should not expect to receive as large a share of the resources in this sector as a younger person. In Great Britain, such understandings have evolved quietly without the need to examine them openly and publicly. Even though the results are not the same, understandings about these matters have developed in the United States as well. Our understandings are, however, that each of us should expect that "everything possible will be done," even if the chances are very small that "everything possible" will have any beneficial effect (Aaron and Schwartz 1984). None of us is ready to accept less for ourselves or those who are near and dear, nor is it likely that providers could or would even be interested in introducing other standards on their own, given the pre-vailing value system and the expected response, starting with private protest and escalating to the threat of legal suits plus public outcry. Thus, any attempt to restrict services must lead to statements specifying the case in opposition to the benefits of treatment. Greater savings in the delivery of health care could be achieved if criteria outlining who should receive maximum care and who should not were determined. In this society such decisions will surely lead to a public debate.

Because specifications regarding who should receive a greater share of health sector resources in the form of more extensive treatment cannot be objectively derived, discussions on such matters require exposition of particularly sensitive values. Few are willing to take the responsibility for initiating discussions stim-ulating public debate regarding values that are at the heart of the social fabric of this society. Such debate certainly risks pitting the younger generation against the older generation; risks blaming the victims of certain types of illnesses for contributing to their own health problems; and risks arguments about social worth involving the moral quality of a person's life, the value of the person's social contribution, innate intelligence, and so on. As long as most of us are not prepared to enter into such discussions or to entrust others to make decisions for us on these matters, one major avenue for achieving savings in the delivery of health care services will remain closed.

THE HEALTH SECTOR FINANCIAL PICTURE

The final characteristic which has played a crucial role in determining the design of the health sector in recent years involves the financial prospects for the future it projects. From one perspective the national economy has been well served by the steady expansion of the health sector for the last ten to fifteen years. Whether the massive medical–industrial complex that has evolved during these years should be greeted as an exciting investment opportunity or as a cause for serious concern regarding potential negative consequences depends on the perspective from which one views this development (Relman 1980). In either case, there is good reason to take seriously the notion that the medical-industrial complex succeeded in the position previously occupied by the military complex (see Table 5). The rise in military expenditures in recent years without any hope that the rate of health expenditures will slow down is at the center of the national budget crisis now plaguing the nation and which, in turn, is responsible for the pressure to cut health care costs.

An obvious solution to this problem has been identified by the nation's policymakers, and attempts are currently underway to implement it, namely, to transfer some portion of the government's share of current health expenditures to the private sector. However, this solution has not been easy to achieve for reasons associated with the size and complexity of this sector. The scenario which has resulted is the following one. The elderly, and others whose health care bills are of catastrophic dimensions, are growing in number; the cost of this type of care constitutes a substantial portion of the government's health care bill; and no one who finds himself or herself in this situation is willing to accept restraints on his or her use of services or increased cost-sharing without a fight. Because so many of those in this situation are both politically aware and well represented, their resistance is formidable. Similarly, the private health insurance industry refuses to assume the burden of cost shifting without making certain its clientele is told that cost shifting from the public portion to the private portion of the health care bill is responsible for the increase in premiums, and many employee benefit packages are being revised as a result. Thus, while the need to control rising costs is a real problem, no one—neither those who consume health services, nor those who deliver health services, nor those who play an intermediate role (providing insurance, supplies, and such)—is willing to accept cuts in his or her particular stake in current health care arrangements. Add to this the difficulty we seem to be having in confronting the fact that a substantial share of the explanation for rising costs is attributable to factors that do not readily lend themselves to the effort to impose cost controls, namely, the growth in the number of persons who utilize health services, the expanded range of medical interventions that are available, and the fact that more seriously ill persons are being treated (Scitovsky and McCall 1976; Scott, Flood, and Ewy 1979).

In recent years we as a society opted for a control system which does not require us to confront these realities. We have chosen to reduce rising health care costs by supporting an approach that would lead to improved efficiency in the operation of the health sector. No one can argue with the goal of reducing inefficiency. To what extent this approach succeeds remains to be seen. The process of selecting measures of success to satisfy the majority of those who have an interest in this sector will be particularly interesting to follow. To illustrate, to the extent that there is a consensus about the steps that will lead to cost savings without risk to health, a reduction in in-patient procedures is without doubt the leading contender. Accordingly, the mechanisms put in place, particulary DRGs, include incentives to encourage the substitution of out-patient care for in-patient care or, at the very least, shorter in-patient stays. (It is interesting that Sloan and Valvona [1986] have concluded that the recent decline in length of stay is due to factors other than the mechanisms associated with market competition.) The effect of the changes taking place has been rapid and extensive enough to have dramatic effects on hospitals, which are undergoing a period of extensive reorganization; some have closed, others have merged, many have entered into contracts with hospital management firms, and so on (Institute of Medicine 1983; Kelly and O'Brien 1983). Although the evidence is not available yet, we should not be surprised if the hospital portion of the health bill, which is the biggest single item, declines. However, the question that must be answered is: Does evidence that this portion is declining, or at minimum not increasing, constitute success? Or is the size of the whole health care bill a better indicator? There are those who argue that it is the "little ticket items" (diagnostic tests) that should be scrutinized (Fineberg 1979). The shift from in-patient to out-patient care may not have a strong effect on this portion of the health care bill. There is also some suspicion that the emphasis on out-patient care may produce increased utilization of out-patient services well beyond the level that could be expected as a result of the shift away from in-patient care, which is to say, increased marketing of out-patient services may induce an increased demand for such services. Whether the increased use of out-patient services is interpreted as desirable depends on whether it is appropriate. Obviously, those who are interested in measuring the effects of recent trends inspired by mechanisms intended to produce cost savings do not face an easy assignment in selecting measures of success that will please everyone.

It will be some time before a consensus can be reached regarding appropriate measures of cost-saving success as well as evaluation techniques to be employed in order to determine the impact that the most recent changes in the organization of the health care delivery system have had. During this time, it is very unlikely that health will decline in worth as a prized social commodity. Accordingly, there is little reason to expect that either personal energy or financial investment will be redirected. In effect, the image this sector projects is imbued with the promise of opportunity in the future. As long as this is true, and as I have said at present there is no reason to believe that this will not be true in the future, investors will continue to put their dollars on what appears to be a safe bet, and individuals will continue to invest their energies in pursuing careers in this sector. As long as this scenario is perceived to be accurate, the health sector will continue to function as a crucial segment in the backbone of the nation's economy. In effect, the nation's economic stability is being buttressed by the confidence that society has in the continued financial viability of the health sector. If this is true, then a severe decline in health expenditures would have negative consequences for the economy as a whole. Perhaps a decline in total health expenditures is not the measure of success we should be using. Perhaps we should be defining cost containment success as reduction in the federal government share of health care costs rather than reduction in health costs as a whole.

DECIDING ON A SYSTEM OF SOCIAL CONTROL

The analogy that comes to mind to illustrate what has been happening in the health sector over the past few decades is that it has fallen into a deep circular rut from which we are now having difficulty extricating it. The circularity of this rut is caused by the following pattern: as each new health sector problem is identified, a mechanism (that is, an agency, incentive program, or such) is created to address it; a sizable number of people become involved in the operations of the mechanism; after a short period of time some faction of observers begins pointing out its shortcomings and proposing alternatives; however, those involved in the operations of that mechanism have a stake in defending it and do so; the rhetoric escalates; those involved in the mechanism's operations eventually start to become demoralized and move into other parts of the health sector; the mechanism begins to wither away from lack of support; meanwhile, the problems that came to light while the mechanism in question was operative are thought to be even more pressing; and a new mechanism is introduced based on the presumed urgency of the need for it, which brings another wave of participants whose interest in the operations of the newest mechanism become quickly vested. And the circular rut begins anew! The rut continues to grow deeper, of course, with the increased weight of each new wave of participants. Finding a way out of this rut, obviously, does not become any easier with delay.

Throughout this discussion I have maintained there are only three options from which to choose in seeking a way out. I will outline the strengths and weaknesses of each, but the list is necessarily short because there are only a few points on which most of us can agree.

According to the literature on organizations, the greatest concern with regard to the administrative approach is its tendency to spawn lumbering, impersonal, and inefficient structures that defeat their own original purposes. In the case of health planning, as is often true of other bureaucratic endeavors, one of the primary purposes is representation of the public interest, which is at risk of being jeopardized by widespread inefficiency. The picture painted of the professional system of control includes equally unattractive features. We are told that professional control systems have a tendency to evolve to benefit the members of the profession. The professionals, in this case physicians, can be expected to devote a large portion of their energies to protecting their rights to perform certain types of work for which they are then in a position to charge high fees. Furthermore, the evidence from the past indicates that there has been little room in this approach to accommodate measures to address the special situation of the poor, whose health is generally worse but who are unable to afford all the health care they need. The flaws in the third approach to control available to us, the market approach, revolve around two basic features. First, the most basic tenet of the market system requires that unprofitable units of an enterprise be identified, and if their profitability cannot be improved they are to be abandoned. The fact that some people depend upon the services provided by such unprofitable units is considered unfortunate but not the responsibility of institutions operating according to market principles. Second, the market approach is based on the idea that consumers are capable of making informed choices, which some critics argue is improbable.

Thus, we are faced with choosing among three approaches to control over the health care delivery system, each of which is clearly imperfect. On the other hand, each also has certain strengths to be considered. The administrative approach is undoubtedly in the best position to assess the overall distribution of health care resources. For one, it is generally agreed that data on the distribution of resources, utilization of services, and perceptions about the availability of health care services are necessary to do planning of any sort; and everyone, except those who are politically conservative in the extreme, agrees that the government should accept primary responsibility for collecting such data. For these reasons, the contribution made by the administrative approach cannot be disregarded.

The most significant characteristic of the administrative approach to control, its stance regarding the role the public should have in determining the kinds of services that will be available, must also be considered. The professional approach is basically silent on this point. The market approach does support the public's right to have a say about the services that will be available; however, the mechanisms it favors differ substantially from those employed by the administrative approach. In a system based on the administrative approach, the public is provided with an open forum where information is shared and options are debated by its representatives. The problems associated with finding appropriate public representatives is where this mechanism falters, as is clear from the literature reviewed in preceding chapters. Those who advocate a system based on market control use this point of weakness to argue that the market approach is superior because it is, by its nature, sensitive to consumer preferences which are expressed as demand for particular kinds of services. Whether one believes this is a superior or inferior mechanism depends on whether one believes that:

1. increased demand will result in an increased supply and ultimately depress the cost of certain services; or
2. that dependence on demand will reduce the access of those who are unable to pay for services that an increasing demand will produce because scarcity rather than an increased supply will be the most likely result. At the heart of this argument is the matter of physician-induced demand and its natural limits.

The key feature of the market approach to control is its emphasis on utilizing practices developed in the private sector intended to increase operating efficiency.

It is interesting that in the relatively short period of time that this approach to control has been in effect in the health sector, it has had sufficient impact to result in evidence that obvious differences between the not-for-profit and for-profit operating styles are no longer apparent. There are some who would argue that this is due to the fact that the profit motive may not have had as much explanatory power as it has been generally credited with by the popular wisdom and by economists (Pattison and Katz 1983; Register, Sharp, and Bivin 1985; Sloan and Valvona 1986; Watt et al. 1986).

Less attention has been directed in recent years to the advantages the professional system of control has to offer. However, one of its undeniable strengths is its commitment to the development of medical science and its application. While advancement in this sector, as in other scientific arenas, can be fostered by directing more funds for research toward one set of research problems rather than another, no one outside of the health sector, or more specifically the medical profession, is in a position to advance medical knowledge because no one else is in a position to verify the benefits of new developments in medical knowledge in practice. In effect, because an equivalent level of knowledge and expertise is required to evaluate or extend the work of others who are developing medical science or applying it in practice, the medical profession has a singular advantage. The health planning legislation (PL 93–641) passed in 1974 provides a particularly good illustration of this. In spite of the fact that the legislative intent was to reduce the influence of providers and increase the influence of consumers in health planning agencies, the authors of this legislation nevertheless had no alternative but to turn to professional expertise in developing the standards that became the regulatory guidelines for evaluating the CON proposals.

THE RHETORIC OF DEBATE

Beyond the fact that the information helpful in clarifying the choices confronting us has not been well organized and readily available is the rhetorical style of current debates about health sector problems and their resolution (Doubilet, Weinstein, and McNeil 1986). The rhetoric of criticism that characterizes such debates, however, should not be taken too literally. This is because so many of the critics who comment on prevailing health care delivery arrangements start by identifying the flaws found in a single mechanism of control and conclude sounding as if all current arrangements are flawed and should be abandoned. While some critics do intend to convey this message, many more probably do not. Whether they intend this or not, however, is a separate issue from the function of the debate itself. Consider the opportunities involved.

If one views the debates about the superiority of one set of mechanisms over another dispassionately, then one can see that the health sector provides a particularly interesting forum for intellectual debate as well as experimentation. The mechanisms that are the products of these debates have a good chance of being implemented and tested in the real world. Thus, it possible to have a part in tinkering with social control mechanisms on a grand scale by creating massive field experiments.

If such a dispassionate view does not strike one as intellectually stimulating but as callous and disruptive, even if not always detrimental to the nation's health, then a revision in the incendiary rhetorical style currently employed by the critics of the mechanisms being used by the health sector might be the first step. The next step might be to identify points of consensus regarding the steps leading to workable solutions. To date far more energy has gone into criticizing alternative approaches and providing a platform for advocating a favorite control mechanism, which has, in turn, more to do with advancing a particular intellectual predisposition, than resolving the problems confronting the health care delivery system.

While it is clearly the business of scholars to engage in vigorous intellectual debate, the consequences of such debates for the operations of the health sector have not been entirely beneficial. The major consequences include a significant loss of public confidence in the health sector, a considerable amount of confusion about alternatives, and the perception that the problems of the health sector are of crisis proportion.

In the end, the rhetoric of criticism realistically can only aim to discredit alternative approaches to control in order to gain an incremental margin of control rather than total control over the health sector. In essence, it is time to acknowledge the fact that all three systems of control are now operative and must continue to coexist in order for the health sector to function.

In sum, we as a society have been reluctant to confront two crucial facts as they relate to the health sector, namely, that no system of control is flawless and that the resources that can be devoted to this sector can no longer be treated as if they were unlimited. Any approach to control that attempts to contain costs in the health sector will of necessity have to confront questions regarding the allocation of resources. However, because each approach takes a different view of this challenge, we must take into consideration the functions each of the three approaches was originally mandated to perform and develop a higher level of consensus regarding the strengths and weaknesses of each before opting for changes in current health care delivery arrangements. To date we have employed an expensive and disorganizing policy of trial and error. This pattern has provided us with certain by-products that have a value in their own right, particularly the sophisticated array of evaluation techniques that have accrued. If it were not for the expense and disorganization involved, we could continue to design and construct massive social experiments and watch them evolve. However, for the sake of the ultimate goal involved—improving the nation's health—it seems to me that it is time to move toward a more cooperative stance focusing on ways to use to best advantage the contributions to planning for the nation's health that each of the three approaches to social control over the health sector can contribute rather than continuing to argue about their failings.

Appendix

The Urban HSA, the case study site, is located in a large metropolitan area with a diverse population and an intricate political structure. The agency's history provides a vivid illustration of the latter observation in that the first attempt at constituting an HSA in this area failed. Those in a position to "designate" (approve) it said it was inappropriately constituted because it was obviously composed of the cronies of the local political establishment. Thus, an entirely new HSA had to be created in 1976, two years after the relevant legislation went into effect. The result is that the Urban HSA was not fully staffed and operative for another year or so. In effect, it had been functioning for about three to four years before the shift in the national social climate occurred that brought with it the anti-regulatory stance espoused by the Reagan administration. This is the point at which I asked the Urban HSA for permission to study it.

The staff members were open and accepting of my interest in their work. The first day I arrived, in January, 1982, I was introduced to the people holding administrative positions. I was assigned to one person, the person responsible for CON reviews, who more or less taught me her job. My intention was to become acquainted with the agency and its work before deciding how to proceed in answering the question that the agency's representatives and I had agreed would be the focus of my research, namely, what have we learned from our experience with health planning?

In order to familiarize myself with the agency's work, I spent approximately two and one-half days per week for the first few months reading material in the files, including documents produced by the state and the region elaborating on the law, the regulations, and statutes; past staff reports; annual reports; and so on. I participated in staff sessions in which incoming CON proposals were reviewed. Finally, I attended the monthly meetings of the CON committee and the governing board. The meetings ran for approximately three to four hours. (Occasionally meetings were canceled if the business at hand could be carried over to the next month.) Additional special meetings were called when special problems warranted them.

After approximately six months of participant observation in the agency's work, I decided to begin interviewing HSA participants. My interview schedule was based on four open-ended questions:

1. How did you happen to become involved with the Urban HSA?
2. Do you feel you represent a particular constituency?
3. If you had to evaluate the HSA's performance on a scale of one through five (five being high), how would you rate it?
4. Knowing what we know now, what could the HSA have done differently?

I used this format because it was non-threatening. I knew there was some concern about my presence when I was introduced during the first monthly CON and governing board meetings that I attended. The sense of threat was confirmed when I asked for an interview appointment. Some respondents nervously asked if I was testing their knowledge; others wanted to know if I was gathering material for an exposé. In one case, at the end of the interview, when I said I was finished with the questions I was prepared to ask, the respondent fell back into her chair and said with a sigh of relief: "That wasn't so bad after all." We then went on to talk for another half-hour about her impressions. There were also those who were quick to insist that I use their names in what I was writing. The result is that I concluded that maintaining a conversational tone and asking respondents to answer in their own words would be the best technique. The interviews generally lasted from about twenty-five minutes to one and one-half hours.

During the first month of my participation, the agency was undergoing some reorganization in its structure due to the substantial decrease in funding. Several committees were being merged, leaving only three active committees: one which reviewed federal grants to agencies in the area; another responsible for drafting the agency's plans, that is, the HSP and the AIP; and one which carried out the CON reviews. In the ongoing reorganization some people were being reassigned to the CON review committee from the committees which were being dissolved. Some new people were just beginning their terms of service.

Approximately one-third of the CON review committee members also held appointments on the executive board. I decided to interview the members of the governing board and the CON committee. The final number of interviews (thirty-three) reflects the fact that some people were serving in both capacities, some had already absented themselves even before their terms of service were officially completed, and others felt too new to discuss the HSA's work with me. Finally, while no one refused to be interviewed, it was virtually impossible to contact a few people, and in two cases repeated efforts to find time for the interviews did not produce success. Five persons fell into this category. Since the participants came and went for various reasons during the twenty months I was involved with the HSA, I did not feel that the population of participants had very clear-cut boundaries. I interviewed virtually everyone who was involved and who agreed to be interviewed. This included three ex-officio participants who did not vote.

While I distinguished between the consumer and provider representatives, this distinction turned out to be less obvious than my preconceptions (based on what I had read and heard in general conversation) had led me to expect. Initially, I was distressed to find that committee voting results were not kept indicating whether the providers or the consumers supported or opposed particular proposals. I found, however, that the level of importance assigned to this distinction was considerably greater than was warranted.

For example, I discovered that one person's designation had been changed from consumer to provider representative when his wife finished her nursing education and became employed as a nurse. When I inquired about this, I was asked, in turn, if I thought that doctors' wives were heavily influenced by their husbands. I agreed that it was likely that they were. Then I was asked if I thought that wives who were health professionals were not as likely to have a similar effect. This was not an issue I wanted to debate, which I quickly realized was precisely the point the agency staff wanted to impress upon me. In another instance, an individual with a great deal of administrative experience was taking some time off after setting up a highly successful health care program. This person was classified as a consumer. If these designations seem arbitrary, it is worth remembering that the selection of appropriate representatives was a problem with which most planning agencies had difficulty.

As I was concluding my stay with the Urban HSA, the HSA administrators were considering a variety of reorganization options—merging with adjacent HSAs, reconstructing the agency as a corporation with a for-profit research arm, developing a related advisory unit which might offer additional funding, and involving major business community leaders and representatives of local health institutions to a greater extent. To the best of my knowledge none of these ideas was implemented. It is my impression that the focus of the Urban HSA's activity has shifted to the development of goals and plans for improving area health care as the number of CON reviews being submitted has declined. It is difficult to know, however, how much attention is being given to these plans by either the public or private health care delivery institutions in the area.

References

Aaron, Henry, and William Schwartz
  1984   *Painful Prescription*. Washington, D.C.: The Brookings Institution.
Addiss, Susan
  1985   "Setting Goals and Priorities: 1984 Presidential Address." *American Journal of Public Health* 75 (Nov.): 1276–1280.
Alford, Robert
  1975   *Health Care Politics*. Chicago: University of Chicago Press.
Altman, Drew
  1978   "The Politics of Health Care Regulation: The Case of the National Health Planning and Resources Development Act." *Journal of Health Politics, Policy and Law* 2 (Winter): 560–580.
———; Richard Greene; and Harvey Sapolsky
  1981   *Health Planning and Regulation: The Decision-Making Process*. Washington, D.C.: American University Programs of Health Administration.
Altman, Stuart
  1984   " 'An Honest Broker' for Fine-Tuning Medicare." *Hospitals* 58 (October 1): 102–105.
Andersen, Ronald; Gretchen Fleming; and Timothy Champney
  1982   "Exploring a Paradox: Belief in a Crisis and General Satisfaction with Medical Care." *Milbank Memorial Fund Quarterly* 60 (Spring): 329–354.
Anderson, Odin
  1985   *Health Services in the United States*. Ann Arbor, Mich.: Health Administration Press.
  1968   *Uneasy Equilibrium*. New Haven, Conn.: College and University Press.
Bauer, Katherine
  1978   *Cost Containment Under PL 93–641*. Harvard University Center for Community Health and Medical Care. Washington, D.C.: Department HEW.
  1977   "Hospital Rate Setting—This Way to Salvation?" *Milbank Memorial Fund Quarterly* 55 (Winter): 117–158.

Bauerschmidt, Alan, and Philip Jacobs
  1985   "Pricing Objectives in Nonprofit Hospitals." *Health Services Research* 20: 153–162.
Barber, Bernard
  1963   "Some Problems in the Sociology of the Professions." *Daedalus* 92: 669–688.
Becker, Howard, et al.
  1961   *Boys in White*. Chicago: University of Chicago Press.
Betz, Michael, and Lenahan O'Connell
  1983   "Changing Doctor–Patient Relationships and the Rise in Concern for Accountability." *Social Problems* 31 (October): 84–95.
Bicknell, William, and Diana Walsh
  1975   "Certification of Need: The Massachusetts Experience." *New England Journal of Medicine* (May 15): 1054–1061.
Biles, Brian; Carl Schramm; and J. Graham Atkinson
  1980   "Hospital Cost Inflation Under Rate-Setting Programs." *New England Journal of Medicine* 303 (September 18): 664–668.
Binstock, Robert
  1969   "Effective Planning through Political Influence." *American Journal of Public Health* 59 (May): 808–813.
Blank, David, and George Stigler
  1957   *The Demand and Supply of Scientific Personnel*. New York: National Bureau of Economic Research.
Blendon, Robert, and Drew Altman
  1984   "Public Attitudes about Health-Care Costs." *New England Journal of Medicine* 311 (August 30): 613–616.
Brown, E. Richard
  1979   *Rockefeller Medicine Men*. Berkeley: University of California Press.
Brown, Lawrence
  1982   *The Political Structure of the Federal Health Planning Program*. Washington, D.C.: The Brookings Institution.
  1981   "Some Structural Issues in the Health Planning Program." In Institute of Medicine, *Health Planning in the United States*. Washington, D.C.: National Academy Press.
Bruhn, John
  1973   "Planning for Social Change: Dilemmas for Health Planning." *American Journal of Health* 63 (July): 602–607.
Bucher, Rue
  1962   "Pathology: A Study of Social Movements Within a Profession." *Social Problems* 10: 40–51.
Building America's Health, 1952–1953
  1953   Volumes 1–5. Washington, D.C.: U.S. Government Printing Office.
Bureau of the Census
  1976   *Historical Statistics of the United States, Part I*. Washington, D.C.: U.S. Department of Commerce.
Bureau of Labor Statistics
  1982   "1981 Weekly Earnings of Men and Women Compared in 100 Occupations." News release, March 7, 1982.

Cain, Henry
1981   "Health Planning in the United States: 1980s--A Protagonist's View." *Journal of Health Politics, Policy, and Law* 6 (Spring): 159–171.
Campion, Frank
1984   *The AMA and U.S. Health Policy Since 1940*. Chicago: Chicago Review Press.
Caplow, Theodore
1982   "Decades of Public Opinion: Comparing NORC and Middletown Data." *Public Opinion* (October/November): 30–31.
1954   *The Sociology of Work*. New York: McGraw-Hill.
Carr-Saunders, A. M.
1933   *The Professions*. New York: Oxford Clarendon Press.
Certificate-of-Need Programs
1978   Prepared by Urban Systems and Engineering and Policy Analysis, Inc. (HRA) 79–14006. Washington, D.C.: Department of Health, Education, and Welfare.
Chayet and Sonnenreich.
1978   *Certificate of Need: An Expanding Regulatory Concept*. Washington, D.C.: Medicine in the Public Interest, Inc.
Checkoway, Barry
1981a   "Consumerism in Health Planning Agencies." In Institute of Medicine, *Health Planning in the United States*. Washington, D.C.: National Academic Press.
1981b   "Consumer Movements in Health in Health Planning." In Institute of Medicine, *Health Planning in the United States*. Washington, D.C.: National Academy Press.
———; Thomas O'Rourke; and David Macrina
1981   "Representation of Providers in Health Planning Boards." *International Journal of Health Sciences* 11:573–581.
Cohodes, Donald
1981   "Interstate Variation in Certificate of Need Programs: A Review and Prospectus." In Institute of Medicine, *Health Planning in the United States*. Washington, D.C.: National Academy Press.
———, Brian Kinkead
1984   *Hospital Capital Formation in the 1980s*. Baltimore: Johns Hopkins University Press.
Colombotos, John
1969   "Physicians and Medicare: A Before-After Study of the Effects of Legislation on Attitudes." *American Sociological Review* 34 (June): 318–334.
Colt, Avery
1970   "Elements of Comprehensive Health Planning." *American Journal of Public Health* 60 (July): 1194–1204.
1969   "Public Policy and Planning Criteria In Public Health." *American Journal of Public Health* 59 (Sept.): 1678–1685.
Committee on Educational Tasks in Comprehensive Health Planning, Public Health Education Section
1970   "A Report on Health Education—Its Relationship to Comprehensive Health

Planning at State Level." *American Journal of Public Health* 60 (April): 751–756.

Curran, William J.
1974   "A National Survey and Analysis of State Certificate of Need Laws for Health Facilities." In Clark Havighurst (ed.), *Regulating Health Facilities Construction*. Washington, D.C.: American Enterprise Institute.
————; Richard Steele; and Ellen Ober
1975   "Government Intervention on Increase." *Hospitals* 49 (May 16): 57–61.

Daniels, Arlene
1973   "How Free Should Professions Be?" In Eliot Friedson (ed.), *The Professions and Their Prospects*. Beverly Hills: Sage.

DeSantis, Grace
1983   "Review Article: Reappraising the Professions." *Sociology of Health and Illness* 5 (July): 220–228.
1980   "Interviewing as Social Interaction." *Qualitative Sociology*, 2 (January): 72–98.

De Solla Price, John
1963   *Little Science, Big Science*. New York: Columbia University Press.

Dingwall, Robert, and Philip Lewis
1983   *The Sociology of the Professions*. New York: St. Martins.

Doubilet, Peter; Milton Weinstein; and Barbara McNeil
1986   "Use and Misuse of the Term Cost 'Effective' in Medicine." *New England Journal of Medicine* 314 (January 23): 253–256.

Downs, George
1981   "Monitoring the Health Planning System: Data, Measurement, and Inference Problems." In Institute of Medicine, *Health Planning in the United States*. Washington, D.C.: National Academy Press.

Dunham, Andrew, and James Morone
1983   *Politics of Innovation: The Evolution of DRG Rate Regulation in New Jersey*. Princeton: Health Research and Education Trust.

Ehrenreich, Barbara and John
1970   *The American Health Empire*. New York: Vintage Books.

Ellenburg, Dorothy
1981   "Special Interests vs. Citizen Control: Who Owns Planning?" In Institute of Medicine, *Health Planning in the United States*. Washington, D.C.: National Academy Press.

Ellwood, Paul
1974   "Models for Organizing Health Services and Implications for Legislative Proposals." In Irving Zola and John McKinlay (eds.), *Organizational Issues in the Delivery of Health Services*. New York: Prodist.

Emerson, Haven
1945   *Local Health Units for the Nation*. New York: The Commonwealth Fund.

Enthoven, Alain
1980   "The Competition Strategy: Status and Prospects." *New England Journal of Medicine* 304 (January 8): 109.

Ermann, M. David
1976   "The Social Control of Organizations in the Health Care Area." *Milbank Memorial Fund Quarterly* 54: 167–183.

Etzioni, Amitai
  1969   *The Semi-Professions and Their Organizations*. New York: The Free Press.
Evans, Robert
  1983   "Incomplete Vertical Integration in the Health Care Industry: Pseudomarkets
          and Pseudopolicies." *Annals* 468: 60–87.
  1974   "Supplier-Induced Demand: Some Empirical Evidence and Implications."
          In Mark Perlman (ed.), *The Economics of Health and Medical Care*. New
          York: John Wiley and Sons.
Ewing, Oscar Ross
  1948   *The Nation's Health, A Ten-Year Program: A Report to the President*. Wash-
          ington, D.C.: U.S. Government Printing Office.
Falk, I. S.; C. R. Rorem; and M. D. Ring
  1933   *The Costs of Medical Care*. Chicago: University of Chicago Press.
Fein, Rashi
  1981   "Preface." *Health Planning in the United States*, vol. I. Washington D.C.:
          National Academy Press.
Feingold, Eugene
  1969   "The Changing Political Character of Health Planning." *American Journal
          of Public Health* 59 (May): 803–808.
Feldstein, Martin
  1981   *Hospital Costs and Health Insurance*. Cambridge, Mass.: Harvard University
          Press.
  1971   *The Rising Cost of Hospital Care*. Washington, D.C.: Information Resources
          Press.
Fifer, Ellen
  1969   "Hang-ups in Health Planning." *American Journal of Public Health* 59
          (May): 765–769.
Fineberg, Harvey
  1979   "Clinical Chemistries: The High Cost of Low Cost Diagnostic Tests." In
          Stuart Altman and Robert Blendon (eds.), *Medical Technology: The Culprit
          Behind Health Care Costs?* Washington, D.C.: Department of Health, Ed-
          ucation, and Welfare.
Flexner, Abraham
  1910   *Medical Education in the United States and Canada*. New York: The Carnegie
          Foundation for the Advancement of Teaching.
Fotion, N.
  1985   "Final Report from a Health Care Planner." *Health Care Management Re-
          view* 10 (Winter): 83–85.
Frazier, Todd
  1970   "The Questionable Role of Statistics in Comprehensive Health Planning."
          American Journal of Public Health, 60 (September): 1701–1705.
Freidson, Eliot
  1970a   *Profession of Medicine*. New York: Dodd, Mead, and Co.
  1970b   *Professional Dominance*. Chicago: Aldine.
  1985   "The Reorganization of the Medical Profession." *Medical Care Review* 42
          (Spring): 11–35.
Friedman, Emily

1984   "Those Wonderful People Who Brought You DRGs." *Hospitals* (March): 81–88.

Fuchs, Victor

1984   "The Rationing of Medical Care." *New England Journal of Medicine* 311 (December 13): 1572–1573.

1974   *Who Shall Live?* Health Economics and Social Choice. New York: Basic Books.

Fuchs, Victor, and Marcia Kramer

1972   *Determinants of Expenditures for Physicians' Services in the United States, 1948–1968.* Rockville, Md: National Bureau of Economic Research.

Galbraith, John Kenneth

1967   *The New Industrial State.* Boston: Houghton Mifflin.

1958   *The Affluent Society.* Boston: Houghton Mifflin.

Gallup, George

1978   *The Gallup Poll, Public Opinion, 1972–1977.* Wilmington, Del.: Scholarly Resources, Inc.

1972   *The Gallup Poll, Public Opinion, 1935–1971.* New York: Random House.

Garceau, Oliver

1941   *The Political Life of the American Medical Association.* Cambridge, Mass.: Harvard University Press.

Ginsburg, Paul, and Frank Sloan

1984   "Hospital Cost Shifting." *New England Journal of Medicine* 310 (April 5): 893–898.

Ginzberg, Eli

1983   "Cost Containment—Imaginary and Real." *New England Journal of Medicine* 308 (May 19): 1220–1224.

1982   "Procompetition in Health Care." *Milbank Memorial Fund Quarterly* 60 (Summer): 386–398.

1969   "Facts and Fancies About Medical Care." *American Journal of Public Health*, 59 (May): 785–794.

Goldsmith, Jeff

1981   *Can Hospitals Survive? The New Competitive Health Care Market.* Homewood, Ill.: Dow Jones-Irwin.

Goode, William

1960   "Encroachment, Charlatanism, and the Emerging Professions: Psychology, Sociology, and Medicine." *American Sociological Review* 25: 902–913.

Gottlieb, Symond

1974   "A Brief History of Health Planning in the United States." In Clark Havighurst (ed.), *Regulating Health Facilities Construction.* Washington, D.C.: American Enterprise Institute.

Greenberg, Warren

1978   *Competition in the Health Care Sector: Past, Present, and Future.* Proceedings of a Conference Sponsored by the Bureau of Economics, Federal Trade Commission. Washington, D.C.: U.S. Government Printing Office.

Greenwood, Ernest

1957   "Attributes of a Profession." *Social Work* 2: 44–55.

Gregg, Alan

1956   *Challenge to Contemporary Medicine*. New York: Columbia University Press.

Gross, Edward
1958   *Work and Society*. New York: Thomas Y. Crowell.

Hall, Oswald
        "The Informal Organization of the Medical Profession." *Canadian Journal of Economic and Political Science* 12 (February): 30–44.

Hall, Thomas
1972   "The Political Aspects of Health Planning." In William Reinke (ed.), *Health Planning: Qualitative Aspects and Quantitative Techniques*. Baltimore: Johns Hopkins University.

Halmos, Paul
1973   "Introduction." In Paul Halmos (ed.), *Professionalisation and Social Change. The Sociological Review Monograph* 20. Keele, Staffordshire: University of Keele.

Harrington, Michael
1962   *The Other America*. New York: Macmillan.

Harris, Louis.
1983   *The Equitable Healthcare Survey*. Conducted for the Equitable Life Assurance Society of the United States (August).

Harris, Louis, and Associates
1983   *The Equitable Healthcare Survey: Options for Controlling Costs*. New York: Equitable Life Assurance Society.

Haug, Marie
1973   "Deprofessionalization: An Alternative Hypothesis for the Future." In Paul Halmos (ed.), *The Sociological Review Monograph* 20. Keele, Staffordshire: University of Keele.
——, and Marvin Sussman
1969   "Professional Autonomy and the Revolt of the Client." *Social Problems* 17 (Fall): 153–161.

Havighurst, Clark
1978   "Professional Restraints in Innovation in Health Care Financing." *Duke Law Journal* (May): 303–307.
1973   "Regulation of Health Facilities and Services by 'Certificate of Need.'" *Virginia Law Review* (October): 1143–1242.

Hellinger, Fred
1976   "The Effect of Certificate of Need Legislation on Hospital Investment." *Inquiry* 13 (June): 187–193.

Hershey, Nathan, and Deborah Robinson
1981   "Health Planning and Certificate of Need: The Quality Dimension." *Health Policy Quarterly* 1 (Winter): 243–268.

Hochbaum, G. M.
1969   "Consumer Participation in Health Planning: Toward Conceptual Clarification." *American Journal of Public Health* 59 (September): 1698–1705.

Hodge, Robert; Paul Siegel; and Peter Rossi
1964   "Occupational Prestige in the United States: 1925–1963." NORC draft of Survey No. 466.

1960   "How Your Earnings Compare." (no author) *Medical Economics* (October 24): 38–47.

Howell, Julianne
1981   *Regulating Hospital Capital Investment: The Experience in Massachusetts.* Washington, D.C.: National Center for Health Services Research (PHS) 81–3298.

Huffman, Leslie
1980   "AMA and Specialty Societies." *American Medical News* (July 25): 4.

Hughes, Everett
1958   *Men and Their Work.* Glencoe, Ill.: Free Press.

Hyman, Herbert
1975   *Health Planning: A Systematic Approach.* Germantown, Md.: Aspen Systems.

Iglehart, John
1984   "Opinion Polls on Health Care." *New England Journal of Medicine* 310 (June 14): 1616–1620.
1982   "The New Era of Prospective Payment for Hospitals." *New England Journal of Medicine* 307 (November 11): 1288–1292.

Immershein, Allen
1981   "American Health Care: Paradigm Structures and the Parameters of Change." In Allen Immershein (ed.), *Challenges and Innovations in U.S. Health Care.* Boulder, Col.: Westview Press.

Institute of Medicine
1984   *The New Health Care for Profit.* Washington, D.C.: National Academy Press.
1981   *Health Planning in the United States.* Washington, D.C.: National Academy Press.
1980   *Health Planning in the United States: Issues in Guideline Development.* Washington, D.C.: National Academy of Sciences.

Janowitz, Morris
1952   *The Community Press in an Urban Setting.* Glencoe, Ill.: Free Press.

Jonas, Steven
1971   "A Theoretical Approach to the Question of 'Community Control' of Health Services Facilities." *American Journal of Public Health* 61 (May): 916–921.

Katz, Arthur
1977   "Capital Financing and Capital Expenditure Controls in Not-for-Profit Hospitals." Unpublished paper, Department of Economics, Harvard University. Reported in Certificate of Need Programs. Washington D.C.: Department HEW.

Keelty, Louis; Mimi Law; Russell Philips, Terence Quirin; and Robert McCleery
1970   *One Life—One Physician.* Washington, D.C.: Center for Study of Responsive Law.

Kelly, Joyce, and John O'Brien
1983   *Characteristics of Financially Distressed Hospitals.* National Center for Health Services Research. Washington D.C.: Department HHS.

Kessel, Reuben
1970   "The AMA and the Supply of Physicians." *Law and Contemporary Problems* 35 (Spring): 267–283.

1958   "Price Discrimination in Medicine." *Journal of Law and Economics* 1 (October): 20–53.

Klarman, Herbert
1978   "Health Planning, Prospects, and Issues." *Milbank Memorial Fund Quarterly* 56 (Winter): 78–112.
1976   "National Policies and Local Planning for Health Services." *Milbank Memorial Fund Quarterly* 54 (Winter): 1–28.

Krause, Elliott
1977   *Power and Illness*. New York: Elsevier.
1973   "Health Planning as a Managerial Ideology." *International Journal of Health Services* 3: 445–463.

Kuhn, Thomas
1970   *The Structure of Scientific Revolutions*. Chicago: University of Chicago Press.

Leffler, Keith
1978   "Physician Licensure: Competition and Monopoly in American Medicine." *Journal of Law and Economics* 22 (April): 165–186.

Lefkowitz, Bonnie
1983   *Health Planning: Lessons for the Future*. Rockville, Md.: Aspen.

Lewin and Associates, Inc.
1975   *Evaluation of the Efficiency and Effectiveness of the Section 1122 Review Process*. Springfield, Va.: U.S. Department of Commerce (September).

Lewis, Oscar
1959   *Five Families*. New York: Basic Books.

Lipsky, Michael, and Morris Lounds
1976   "Citizen Participation and Health Care: Problems of Government Induced Participation." *Journal of Health Politics, Policy, and Law* 1 (Spring): 85–111.

Little, Arthur, Inc.
1982   *Development of an Evaluation Methodology for Use in Assessing Data Available to the Certificate of Need (CON) and Health Planning Programs*. Prepared for Department of H.H.S., Cambridge, Mass.

Lortie, Dan
1958   "Anesthesia: From Nurses' Work to Medical Specialty." In E. Gartly Jaco (ed.), *Patients, Physicians, and Illness*. Glencoe, Ill.: Free Press.

Luft, Harold, and Gary Frisvold
1979   "Decision-making in Regional Health Planning Agencies." *Journal of Health Politics, Policy, and Law* 4 (Summer): 250–272.

McCarthy, Carol
1977   "Planning for Health Care." In Steven Jonas (ed.), *Health Care Delivery in the United States*. New York: Springer.

McClure, Walter
1981   "Structure and Incentive Problems in Economic Regulation of Medical Care." *Milbank Memorial Fund Quarterly* 59 (Spring): 107–144.

McIlrath, Sharon
1985   "Effects of PPS on Quality of Care Studied." *American Medical News* (December 27): 2, 27.
1984   "Officials Fear Rush by Voters to All-Payer Rate-Setting Plans." *American Medical News* (November 9): 1, 41.

MacStravic, Robin
   1977   "Size and Performance of Planning Agencies." *Health Services Research* 12 (Summer): 163–173.
Marmor, Theodore, and James Morone
   1980   "Representing Consumer Interests: Imbalanced Markets, Health Planning, and the HSAs." *Milbank Memorial Fund Quarterly* 58 (Winter): 125–165.
Mattison, Berwyn
   1967   "New Horizons—Comprehensive Health Planning for Health." *American Journal of Public Health* 57 (March): 392–400.
Mead, Lawrence
   1977   "Health Policy: The Need for Governance." *Annals* 434 (November): 39–57.
Mellor, Earl
   1985   "Weekly Earnings in 1983: A Look at More than 200 Occupations." 108 *Monthly Labor Review* (January): 54–59.
Moore, Mary
   1971   "The Role of Hostility and Militancy in Indigenous Community Health Advisory Groups." *American Journal of Public Health* 61 (May): 922–930.
Moore, Wilbert
   1970   *The Professions, Roles and Rules*. New York: Russell Sage Foundation.
Morone, James
   1981a   "Models of Representation: Consumers and the HSAs." In Institute of Medicine, *Health Planning in the United States*. Washington, D.C.: National Academy Press.
   1981b   "The Real World of Representation: Consumers and the HSAs." In Institute of Medicine, *Health Planning in the United States*. Washington, D.C.: National Academy Press.
Mott, Basil
   1977   "The New Health Planning System." In Arthur Levin (ed.), *Health Services: The Local Perspective*. New York: Academy of Political Science.
   1969   "The Myth of Planning Without Politics." *American Journal of Public Health* 59 (May): 797–803.
Mott, Peter; Anthony Mott; Jonathan Rudolf; Edward Lane, and Robert Berg
   1976   "Difficult Issues in Health Planning, Development, and Review." *American Journal of Public Health* 66 (August): 473–476.
Navarro, Vicente
   1976   *Medicine Under Capitalism*. New York: Prodist.
National Opinion Research Center
   1984   *General Social Surveys, 1972–1984: Cumulative Codebook. NORC* (July): 152–155.
   1947   *National Opinion on Occupations. Final Report NORC*. University of Denver, April 22.
Newhouse, Joseph
   1981   "The Erosion of the Medical Marketplace." In R. Scheffler (ed.), *Advances for Health Economics and Health Services Research*. Greenwich, Conn.: JAI Press.
O'Conner, John

1974   "Comprehensive Health Planning: Dreams and Realities." *Milbank Memorial Fund Quarterly* 52 (Fall): 143–165.

Owens, Arthur
1984   "Are You Still Losing Out to Inflation?" *Medical Economics* (September 17, 1984): 180–190.
1981   "How's Inflation Treating You?" *Medical Economics* (September 28, 1981): 173–185.
1970   "Inflation Closes in on Physicians' Earnings." *Medical Economics* (December 21, 1970): 63–71.

Palmer, Alan
1979   "Regulation, Professional Responsibility, and Market Forces in the Health Care Field." *Journal of Medical Education* 54 (April): 275–283.

Parker, Alberta
1970   "The Consumer as Policy-Maker—Issues of Training." *American Journal of Public Health* 60 (November): 2139–2153.

Parkinson, C. Northcote
1957   *Parkinson's Law*. Boston: Houghton Mifflin.

Parsons, Talcott
1951   *The Social System*. New York: Free Press.

Pattison, Robert, and Hollie Katz
1983   "Investor-Owned and Not-For-Profit Hospitals." *New England Journal of Medicine* 309 (August 11): 347–353.

Pauly, Mark
1980   *What Now, What Later, What Never?* Washington, D.C.: American Enterprise Institute.

Peterson, Paul
1967   "The Impact of Recent Federal Legislation on Personal Health Services." *American Journal of Public Health* 57 (July): 1091–1099.

"Physicians' Economic Status."
1944   *Medical Economics* (November): 48–49.

"Physicians' Incomes."
1940   *Medical Economics* (September): 38–48.

Polk, Lewis
1909   "Areawide Comprehensive Health Planning: The Philadelphia Story." *American Journal of Public Health* 59 (May): 760–764.

President's Commission for the Study of Ethical Problems in Medicine and Biomedical and Behavioral Research
1982   *Making Health Care Decisions*. Washington, D.C.: U.S. Government Printing Office.

"PRO Rules Criticized for Emphasis on Cost."
1983   *American Medical News* (September 16): 2, 10.

"Public Expresses Increased Concern Over Cost of Care."
1984   *American Medical News* (January 27): 21.

Raab, G. Gregory
1981   "National/State/Local Relationships in Health Planning: Interest Group Reaction and Lobbying." In Institute of Medicine, *Health Planning in the United States*. Washington, D.C.: National Academy Press.

Rayack, Elton

1967   *Professional Power and American Medicine: The Economics of the American Medical Association*. Cleveland: World Publishing Co.

Reeves, Philip
1972   "Data for Health Planning." *American Journal of Public Health* 62 (June): 874–876.

———, David Bergwall; and Nina Woodwide
1979   *Introduction to Health Planning*. Washington, D.C.: Information Resources Press.

Register, Charles; Ansel Sharp; and David Bivin
1985   "Profit Incentives and the Hospital Industry: Are We Expecting Too Much?" *Health Services Research* 20 (June): 225–241.

Reinhardt, Uwe
1981   "The GMENAC Forecast: An Alternative View." *American Journal of Public Health* 71 (October): 1149–1157.

Reiss, Albert
1955   "Occupational Mobility of Professional Workers." *American Sociological Review* (December): 693–700.

Rice, George
1972   "Use of Groups, Councils, and Committees in Comprehensive Health Planning—Birmingham, Alabama Style." *American Journal of Public Health* 62 (July): 977–979.

Richards, Glenn
1984   "Business Examines Hospitals." *Hospitals* 58 (January 1): 61–69.

Richardson, William
1934   "Our Post-Depression Incomes." *Medical Economics* (April): 12–15, 77–81.

Ritzer, George
1977   *Working*. Englewood Cliffs, N. J.: Prentice-Hall.

Roethlisberger, Fritz, and W. J. Dickson
1938   *Management and the Worker*. Cambridge, Mass.: Harvard University Press.

Roseman, April
1972   "Problems and Prospects for Comprehensive Health Planning." *American Journal of Public Health* 62 (January): 16–19.

Russell, Louise
1979   *Technology in Hospitals: Medical Advances and Their Diffusion*. Washington. D.C.: The Brookings Institution.

Salkever, David, and Thomas Bice
1977   "Impact of State Certificate-of-Need Laws on Health Care Costs and Utilization." DHEW Publication No. (HRA) 77–3163.
1976   "The Impact of Certificate-of-Need Controls on Hospital Investment." *Milbank Memorial Fund Quarterly* 54 (Spring): 185–214.

Sapolsky, Harvey
1981   "Bottoms Up Is Upside Down." In Institute of Medicine, *Health Planning in the United States*. Washington, D.C.: National Academy Press.

Schwebel, Andrew; Richard Kershaw; Susan Reeve; John Harung; and William Reeve
1973   "A Community Organization Approach to Implementation of Comprehensive Health Planning." *American Journal of Public Health* 63 (August): 675–680.

Scitovsky, Anne, and Nelda McCall
  1976   *Changes in the Costs of Treatment of Selected Illnesses, 1951–1964–1971.* Washington, D.C.: Department of Health, Education, and Welfare.
Scott, W. Richard; Ann Barry Flood; and Wayne Ewy
  1979   "Organizational Determinants of Services, Quality, and Costs of Care in Hospitals." *Milbank Memorial Fund Quarterly* 57 (Spring): 234–264.
Sheldon, Alan
  1975   *Organizational Issues in Health Care Management.* New York: Spectrum Publications.
Shortell, Stephen; Michael Morrisey; and Douglas Conrad
  1985   "Economic Regulation and Hospital Behavior: The Effects on Medical Staff Organization and Hospital–Physician Relationships." *Health Services Research* 20 (December): 597–628.
Sloan, Frank, and Roger Feldman
  1978   "Competition Among Physicians." In Warren Greenberg (ed.), *Competitions in the Health Care Sector: Past, Present, and Future.* Proceedings of a Conference Sponsored by the Bureau of Economics, Federal Trade Commission. Washington, D.C.: U.S. Government Printing Office.
———, and Joseph Valvona
  1986   "Why Has Hospital Length of Stay Declined? An Evaluation of Alternative Theories." *Social Science and Medicine* 22: 63–73.
Smigel, Erwin
  1954   "Trends in Occupational Sociology in the United States: A Survey of Postwar Research." *American Sociological Review* 19 (August): 398–404.
———, Joseph Monane; Robert Wood; and Barbara Nye
  1963   "Occupational Sociology: A Re-examination." *Sociology and Social Research* 47 (April): 472–477.
Smith, Tom
  1981   "Can We Have Confidence in Confidence? Revisited." In Denis Johnston (ed.), *Measurement of Subjective Phenomena.* Washington, D.C." U.S. Bureau of the Census.
Somers, Anne, and Herman Somers
  1977   *Health and Health Care.* Germantown, Md.: Aspen Systems Corp.
Somers, Dixie
  1974   Occupational Rankings for Men and Women by Earnings." *Monthly Labor Review* 97 (August): 34–51.
Starr, Paul
  1982   *The Social Transformation of American Medicine.* New York: Basic Books.
Stebbins, Ernest, and Kathleen Williams
  1972   "History and Background of Health Planning in the United States." In William Reinke and Kathleen Williams (eds.), *Health Planning: Qualitative Aspects and Quantitative Techniques.* Baltimore: The Johns Hopkins Press.
Stevens, Rosemary
  1971   *American Medicine and the Public Interest.* New Haven: Yale University Press.
Stiles, Samuel
  1983   *Briefing Paper on Certificate of Need.* Bethseda, Md.: Alpha Center.
Strauss, Marvin, and Ida DeGroot

1971   "A Bookshelf on Community Planning for Health." *American Journal of Public Health* 61 (April): 656–679.

Stroman, Duane

1979   *The Quick Knife*. Port Washington, N.Y.: Kennikat Press.

Tannen, Lewis

1980   "Health Planning as a Regulatory Strategy: A Discussion of Its History and Current Uses." *International Journal of Health Services* 10: 115–130.

Thurow, Lester Carl

1985   "The Dishonest Economy." *New York Review of Books* 32 (November 21): 34–37.

1984   "Learning to Say 'No.' " *New England Journal of Medicine* 311 (December 13): 1569–1570.

"Training for Citizen–Consumer Participation in Comprehensive Health Planning."

n.d.   *Final Report*. Center for Continuing Education. University of Chicago.

Vladek, Bruce

1985   "The Dilemma Between Competition and Community Service." *Inquiry* 22 (Summer): 115–121.

1981   "The Market vs. Regulation: The Case for Regulation." *Milbank Memorial Fund Quarterly* 59 (Spring): 209–223.

1977   "Interest-Group Representation and the HSAs: Health Planning and Political Theory." *American Journal of Public Health* 67 (January): 23–29.

Watt, J. Michael; Robert Derzon; Steven Renn; Carl Schramm; James Hahn; and George Pillari

1986   "The Comparative Economic Performance of Investor-Owned Chain and Not-For-Profit Hospitals." *New England Journal of Medicine* 314 (January 9): 89–96.

Wennberg, John; Klein McPherson; and Philip Caper

1984   "Will Payment Based on Diagnosis-Related Groups Control Hospital Costs?" *New England Journal of Medicine* 311 (August 2): 295–300.

——; Benjamin Barnes; and Michael Zubkoff

1982   "Professional Uncertainty and the Problem of Supplier-Induced Demand." *Social Science and Medicine* 16: 811–824.

West, Jonathan and Michael Stevens

1976   "Comparative Analysis of Community Health: Transition from CHPs to HSAs." *Journal of Health Politics, Policy and Law* 1 (Summer): 173–195.

White, Jane See

1982   "Are Specialty Societies Taking Over Organized Medicine?" *Medical Economics*. (May 10): 225, 228.

Wildavsky, Aaron

1979   *Speaking Truth to Power: The Art and Craft of Policy Analysis*. Boston: Little, Brown.

1977   "Doing Better and Feeling Worse: The Political Pathology of Health Policy." *Daedalus* 106 (Winter): 105–123.

Wilensky, Harold

1964   "The Professionalization of Everyone?" *American Journal of Sociology* 70 (September): 137–158.

Woods, David

1986   "Ontario Physicians Fighting Back." *American Medical News* (February 7): 28.

Yoder, Franklin, and Shirley Reed

1970   "Cook County Hospital Facilities and the State Health Department." *American Journal of Public Health* 60 (September): 1706–1711.

"Your Economic Weather Vane."

1952   *Medical Economics* (December): 71–87.

Zubkoff, Michael; Ira Raskin; and Ruth Hanft

1978   *Hospital Cost Containment: Selected Notes for Future Policy.* New York: Prodist.

Zuckerman, Howard

1983   "Industrial Rationalization of a Cottage Industry: Multi-Institutional Hospital Systems." *Annals* 468 (July): 216–230.

Zwick, Daniel

1978   "Initial Development of National Guidelines for Health Planning." *Public Health Reports* 93 (October): 407–420.

Index

About the Author

GRACE BUDRYS is Director of the Public Services Program and Associate Professor of Sociology at DePaul University, Chicago, Illinois. She has contributed articles to *Social Science and Medicine* and *Journal of Health and Illness.*